Nature Has the Cure
Volume 3

Marie Lasater

CONTENTS

i

ACKNOWLEDGMENTS

I'd like to thank the following authors whose contributions were invaluable to this book: Tamara Glascock, Herbalist extraordinaire and Candice Schwien, a true woman of virtue and wisdom

This book is dedicated to my late husband Brad North, without whose loving support and encouragement I would never have been able to achieve my goals over the past 10 years.

1 NIACIN – THE OVERLOOKED VITAMIN

In the field known as orthomolecular medicine, niacin is a super star. For those not familiar with the term, orthomolecular scientists believe that for every disease, there is a corresponding natural cure. Niacin, also known as Vitamin B3 and nicotinic acid, is found in many native plants and has been linked to over 500 biochemical reactions in the body.

Many people have been prescribed Niacin by their physician in order to support their heart by improving vascular flow. Some of the little known effects of niacin include its effects on mental disorders, including bipolar disorder and schizophrenia.

So where do we find this powerful substance in nature? Among native plants in Missouri, finger millet, black cherries, fiddleheads and Jerusalem Artichoke are great sources.

Niacin deficiency

Although it is rarely seen in our society, the disease pellagra is due to niacin deficiency and is marked by severe skin lesions and behavioral problems. Health care providers have a mnemonic to aid in diagnosis: diarrhea, dementia and dermatitis, symptoms that rapidly improve when the patient is treated with niacin. Pellagra was a problem in the 1930s and 1940s, but was essentially eradicated in the United States with addition of niacin to flour.

Schizophrenia a niacin deficiency?

According to Dr. Abram Hoffer, author of the book *Niacin: The Real Story*, schizophrenia is a severe case of pellagra, and can be treated with niacin. It is a well-known fact that niacin deficiency presents with many types of psychiatric symptoms. Current studies are seeking to determine types of schizophrenia most responsive to treatment with niacin. Many schizophrenics don't experience the characteristic skin flush with high niacin doses, indicating they have resistance to the vitamin. Indeed, when these patients are treated with niacin, they are given doses at up to 50 times the recommended daily allowance before improvement is noted.

Alcoholism and niacin deficiency

One of the consequences of excessive and prolonged use of alcohol is mild-to-severe form of pellagra (i.e., some combination of diarrhea, dermatitis, dementia, and possibly death). Nutrition problems in alcoholics start with the replacement of normal calories from food with alcohol, leading to malnutrition and liver damage.

Several studies have described the clinical effectiveness of vitamin B 3 treatment for compulsive drinking behavior, alcohol withdrawal delirium, and for supporting sobriety. Dr. Abram Hoffer, who has studied alcoholism and its treatment extensively has said, "I have been able to bring many alcoholics with severe tremor out of the tremor very quickly by giving them one gram of nicotinic acid only, by mouth. This has helped several alcoholics to terminate a severe alcoholic bout." In his studies, recovery from delirium tremor occurred in 24 hrs. to 4 days in the severe cases. Mr. Bill Wilson, the cofounder of Alcoholics Anonymous (AA), met Abram Hoffer in 1958. Wilson became a strong supporter of niacin in the treatment of alcoholism, and wanted every alcoholic to take vitamin B3 as part of his or her AA experience. He felt they should take niacin at least until they had 6 months of sobriety.

Niacin and cholesterol management

Niacin has a key role in managing cholesterol. Several studies have concluded that it decreases the risk of coronary heart disease and hardening of the arteries by decreasing serum total cholesterol and LDL (bad) cholesterol while raising the level of HDL (good) cholesterol.

Side effects

If you have ever taken niacin in a sizable dose, you are familiar with the "flush," a feeling of warmth, and even reddened skin when the blood vessels dilate. No deaths have ever been attributed to taking too much niacin, but experiencing "the flush" indicates that the body is saturated, so is a signal the dose should be lowered.

2 HERD IMMUNITY?

With the recent case of the mumps (in a previously vaccinated individual) here in Texas County, you may have encountered the term "herd immunity." Those in favor of vaccination describe it as follows: herd immunity is a form of immunity that occurs when the vaccination of a significant portion of a population (or herd) provides a measure of protection for individuals who have not developed immunity. It is thought that when a high percentage of the population is protected through vaccination against a virus or bacteria, it is difficult for a disease to spread because there are so few susceptible people left to infect. Herd immunity is specifically thought to protect those that cannot be vaccinated, such as those with impaired immunity.

Those in favor of vaccination feel that when immunization rates fall, herd immunity can break down, leading to an increase in the number of new cases of a specific disease. One problem with this theory is that over the past 2 years, at least half of new cases of diseases such as mumps and measles occur in previously vaccinated individuals.

The term *Herd Immunity* was actually coined by A.W. Hedrich, an early epidemiologist who studied measles in the USA between 1900 – 1931. He concluded that when 68% of children became immune to measles **due to active infection**, measles epidemics ceased. Unlike vaccines, disease conferred immunity usually lasts a lifetime. As each new generation of children contracted the infection, the immunity of those previously infected was renewed due to their continual re-exposure to the disease, thus maintaining "herd immunity" at all times.

When the measles vaccine was introduced in 1963 with the goal of 100% vaccination, officials were confident that measles would be eradicated in 4 years. Due to the subsequent loss of natural immunity, new dates for eradication were extended to 1982, 2000, and 2010.

Today, a consortium of 180 physicians have concluded that "the eradication of measles would today appear to be an unrealistic goal." As early as 1984, Prof. D. Levy of Johns Hopkins University concluded "if current practices of suppressing natural immunity continue, by the year 2050 a large part of the population will be at risk, and there could be in theory over 25,000 fatal cases of measles in the USA."

Some researchers feel the increase in the outbreaks of Shingles in age 50+ persons correlates with increased chicken pox vaccinations, due to less boosting of immunity by the body to the varicella virus. The chicken pox vaccine is effective in its prevention, but the incidence of shingles in older persons has definitely increased as they are not being re-exposed to the disease, removing a natural booster to immunity.

Before vaccines, infants received antibodies against disease from their mothers who had themselves been infected as children and re-exposed to disease in the course of their lifetime. Today's babies born to vaccinated mothers never exposed to disease do not receive these natural antibodies, making them more vulnerable to disease.

3 MUCUNA – PAIN RELIEF AND MORE

Dioclea grandiflora is a genus of plants in the pea family, native to North and South America. Commonly called Mucuna, the plant is the subject of much medical research. Like many natural remedies, it can by found on Amazon.com where it is promoted as a source of Dopamine, improving mood and relaxation, and also an adjunct treatment for Parkinson's disease. The seeds of this plant in the pea family are buoyant drift seeds, dispersed by rivers. It is a tall climbing plant, with leaves composed of three small oblong leaflets and large seeds.

Mucuna is a potential source of compounds containing medicinal effects. The plant is a popular subject in the search for new drugs of natural origin. In traditional medicine, an infusion of the roots from the plant is used to treat prostate disorders and kidney stones and also for its effects on the central nervous system. Several studies have revealed that the plant has pain relieving, cardiovascular, antioxidant and anti-inflammatory activities. Flavonoids are the major constituents of Mucuna that account for most of the pharmacological properties so far discovered.

Nervous System

A 2013 study looked at the nervous system effect of Mucuna, using the pods of the plant. Researchers examining the anxiety, depressant, and anti-seizure effects found that there was a depressant effect on the nervous system, and also an anti-anxiety effect.

Another study in 2010 utilized the stem bark from the plant and found increased protection against seizures, decreased anxiety, and longer periods of sleep.

Pain Relief

The plant Mucuna has two components, dioflorin and dioclenol, that help in pain relief. In a 1997 study, an extract from the root bark was collected and administered to laboratory animals. Dioflorin had an effect on pain similar to that of Morphine, and dioclenol also had pain-relieving affects.

Sleep

Mucuna does support sleep, but researchers have found that doses of 342 and 685 mg/kg are required to see any effect.

Vasorelaxant

A flavonoid isolated from the roots of Dioclea grandiflora (Mucuna), was tested for vasorelaxant activity. The plant proved to have vasorelaxant effects on the aorta, an effect that could be beneficial to the heart.

Nutrition

Although mucuna is in the legume family, and is a source of protein, it has been found to have poor digestibility, and is not a good nutritional choice. Several studies have investigated its use as a famine food, but due to side effects, it probably shouldn't be consumed as a food. In addition, lectins found in the seeds bind with carbohydrates, limiting their absorption and leading to dietary deficiencies.

Side Effects

Data in the literature show that adverse reactions like dermatitis, palpitations, headache and hallucinations were observed in humans after consuming seeds from the plant.

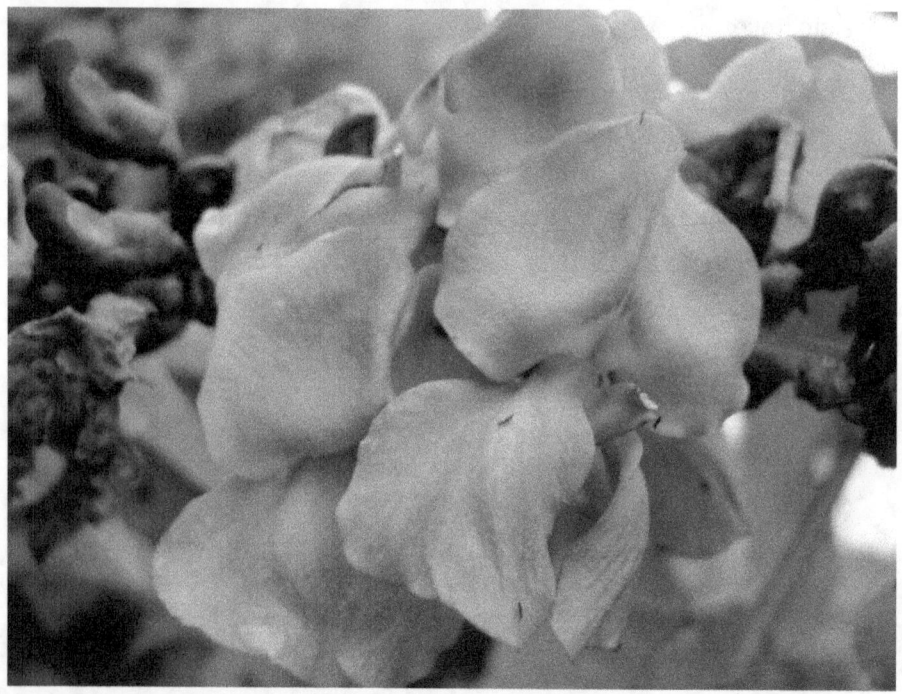

Mucuna is a plant in the pea family, native to North and South America.

4 EUCALYPTUS

Eucalyptus is not native to Missouri, but is still a valuable medicinal plant that can be grown here. The medicinal properties are obtained from oil extracted from the leaves and branch tips, and also from dried leaves. The eucalyptus genus includes hundreds of species of trees and shrubs, all in the myrtle family. The plant is very common in Australia. Like other members of the myrtle family, eucalyptus leaves are covered with oil glands, and exudes a fresh, pleasant fragrance.

Eucalyptus is not frost tolerant, so it is best to grow it in a container that can be brought inside during the winter. It grows very quickly, so choose a large pot! Never allow the plant to go completely dry, or it will shrivel and die. Although it remains evergreen, your tree will naturally shed a lot of leaves; these can be collected and used later. Eucalyptus should be kept separated from other plants, as they release compounds that inhibit nearby plant growth, a quality that has proven helpful in treating and preventing the spread of influenza.

Joint Pains

Eucalyptus is a key ingredient in a spray medication called "Eezpain" that has been studied for its pain relieving and anti-inflammatory properties. In a study published in 2015, when the spray was applied to knee and wrist joints, neck and shoulder, forearms and lower back, 20 subjects reported significant pain relief.

Eucalyptus oil is thought to prevent pain by blocking pain receptors. Eucalyptol, one of the components found in eucalyptus, blocks the production of prostaglandins (pain-causing chemicals) in the same way as aspirin.

Antibacterial properties

In developing countries where antibiotics can be too expensive and out of the reach of many people, plant sources are often used for their germ-killing properties. Eucalyptus is one of these, and has studied for use against a prevalent bacteria, *Staph aureus*. Different concentrations of both dried and fresh Eucalyptus leaves were used to complete a study published in 2016, and it was found that fresh leaves are more effective than dried leaves in treating infection.

Antifungal properties

A 2016 study compared the anti-fungal effect of eucalyptus and the common anti-fungal drug Nystatin. Eucalyptus was effective as an antifungal, although not to the extent of Nystatin. Where pharmaceuticals are not available, Eucalyptus remains an effective treatment for common fungal infections such as Athlete's Foot.

Nail fungus is a common disease that accounts for half of all nail issues. It is largely undertreated, and can cause progressive destruction of the nail, with age increasing frequency of infection and potential for complications. In a 2015 study, the nails of 22 people with a total of 70 infected toenails with nail fungus infection were treated with eucalyptus. Nails with superficial infection were found to have 86% clearance of infection after four months, while up to 50% of all nails with more severe infection were beginning to show a zone of clearance as the nail grew out. Researchers concluded eucalyptus oil is more effective as an antifungal treatment for fungal infected, and may provide an acceptable and cheaper alternative to prescription topical antifungal agents.

Scabies

A 2016 study looked at eucalyptus oil as an alternative treatment for scabies. When several different essential oils were compared, tea tree oil, clove oil, palmarosa oil and eucalyptus oil were found most effective in treating scabies infections in humans and animals, in addition to controlling the mites in the environment.

Blood Pressure

Inhaling eucalyptus oil has been shown to reduce blood pressure. This was investigated in a 2013 study that looked at the effect of eucalyptus on pain and blood pressure after total knee replacement. The autonomous nervous system is affected by smell, so inhaling essential oil can have a direct action on the nervous system. It has been found to decrease blood pressure by relaxing arteries. In the study, systolic blood pressure (the top number) was found to be significantly lower after inhalation of eucalyptus, but the inhalation had no effect on diastolic (the bottom number) or pulse. Inhalation of 3% eucalyptus oil every 30 minutes for 3 days after total knee replacement effectively reduced pain and inflammatory responses. This study showed that eucalyptus oil inhalation was effective in reducing patient's subjective pain and blood pressure after surgery.

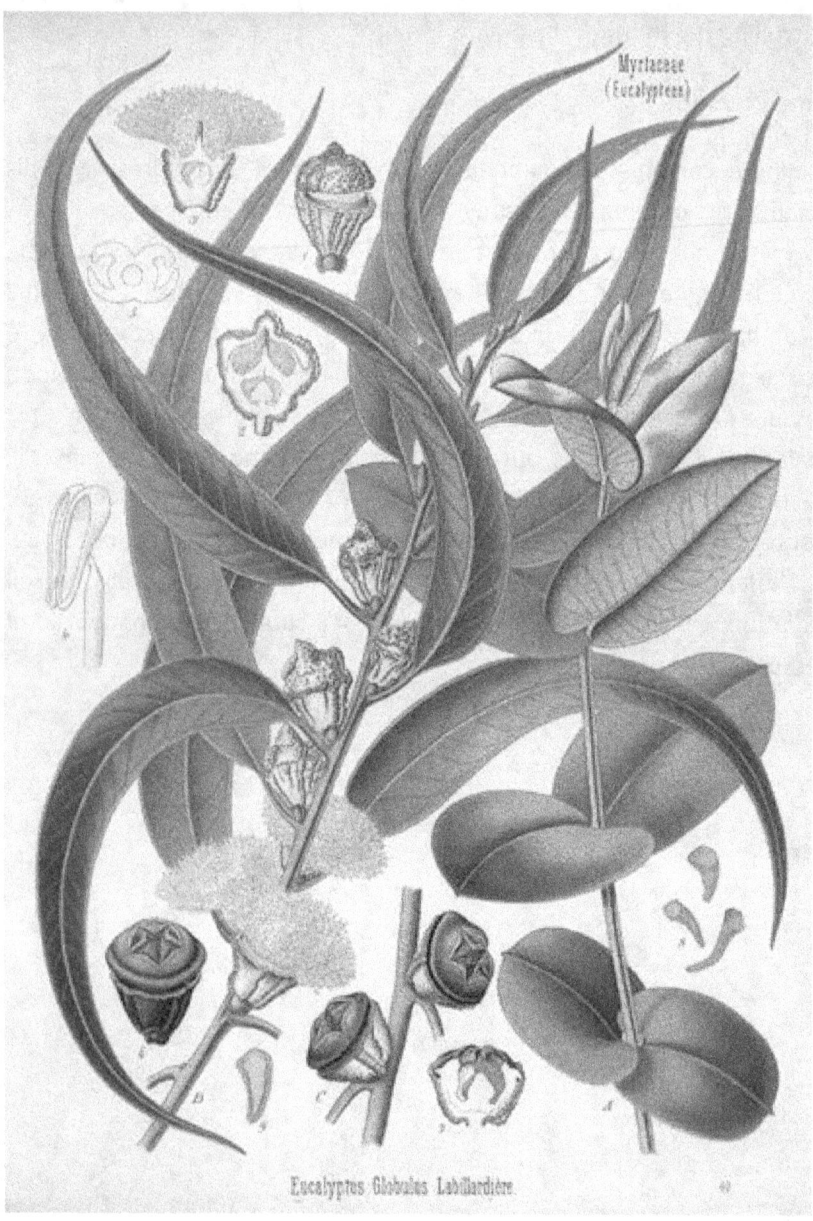

Medicinal properties of eucalyptus are obtained from oil extracted from the leaves and branch tips, and also from dried leaves

4 MOUSE EAR (HAWKWEED)

Mouse Ear (Pilosella officinarum) is native to Europe and parts of Asia, but can be found in North America and is present in Missouri. It is easy to recognize and resembles the dandelion, but with flowers of a lighter yellow and mouse-ear shaped leaves. Flowers appear between May and September, with a single flower on each stalk of the plant. The hair-covered leaves grow close to the ground. The plant prefers dry, sandy soil, and is considered a weed. Wildlife grazes on the plant and can help to prevent overgrowth. The best time to harvest the plant is when it is flowering. The mouse ear plant produces stolons, horizontal branches that give rise to new rosettes at the extremity of the plant. Every rosette on the plant is able to grow into a new genetic copy, making it potentially invasive. Mouse ear can also be grown from seeds.

Use in Respiratory Conditions

While the seeds for the plant are available for purchase online, mouse ear has fallen out of common use as a medicinal agent. It can be taken by mouth to treat wheezing, asthma, bronchitis, coughs, and whooping cough. A poultice can be applied to wounds. When taken by mouth, mouse ear is much less bitter than other plants in its category. During the middle ages, when it was called by its Latin name Auricula muris, it was commonly used to make an drink used as a tonic, and for its sweat producing and expectorant properties. As a treatment for respiratory problems, this herb soothes the muscles of the bronchial tubes, encourages the cough impulse and also decreases mucus production.

Other Uses

There are also reports of the plant being used to treat diarrhea and liver disease. It has also been used as a home remedy to treat fever, and is also a strong diuretic. Mouse ear contains a component called umbelliferone, a chemical compound that absorbs ultraviolet light and is found in many sunscreens.

External Application

When applied to a wound, the dried leaves help to stop bleeding, and when applied to hemorrhoids, help to shrink swollen tissues. A powder made from dried leaves can be applied nasally to stop nosebleeds.

Dosage

Mouse ear is usually prepared as a tea or a tincture when taken by mouth. To make a tea, add 2 teaspoons of dehydrated leaves to a cup of boiling water, allowing steeping for 10 – 15 minutes. For coughs or other respiratory problems, you can drink it 3 times daily.

To make a tincture

Put 4 ounces of fresh or dried chopped mouse ear leaves into a pint jar; add enough alcohol to cover (such as vodka). Vinegar can be substituted for alcohol, but doesn't possess the same ability to extract the medicinal components of the plant. Use a butter knife along the edge of the jar to remove any air bubbles. Keep in a cool, dark area for at least 8 days, shaking the jar daily. After about 2 weeks, strain the mixture into a dark glass bottle (preferably) through a cheesecloth. If you plan to store for a long period, you can cap the bottle with paraffin wax. The tincture prepared from mouse ear can be taken in dosage of 1 ml to 4 ml 3 times daily. (Note: There are 5 ml in one teaspoon.)

Precautions

Mouse ear contains a blood-thinning component, so should be used with caution in those on blood thinners.

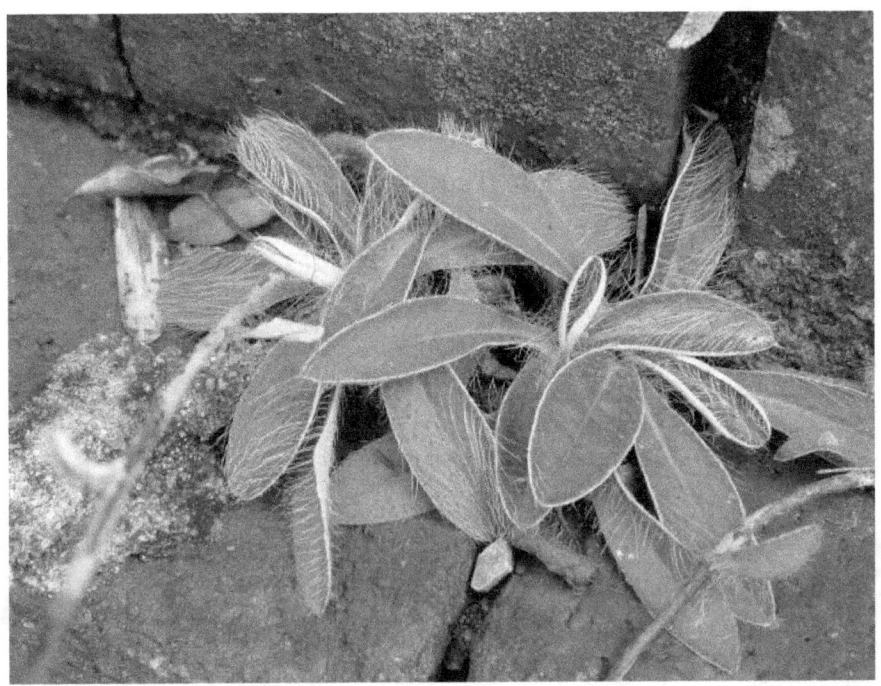

Mouse ear is easy to recognize and resembles the dandelion, but with lighter yellow flowers and mouse-ear shaped leaves.

6 THE HEALING POWER OF PRAYER

Most people have experienced God's healing power. Many of us know several people just this week who have requested our prayers. We stop, we become still, and send our prayers and positive intentions, lifting up those who need healing. Prayer is widely acknowledged in both ancient and modern times as an intervention for alleviating illness and promoting good health

But how does prayer work? What role does it have in our natural healing arsenal? Hundreds of studies have been done attempting to validate specific medical evidence of the effect of prayer. Such research is problematic, for God is the one who heals in response to prayer, but scientists are limited to the study of events in the natural world. In this article, we will discuss some of the recent studies concerning prayer and healing.

Types of prayer

There are several types of prayer. A prayer of transaction is a personal dialogue with God, and a form of submission, in which a person bares their soul, giving it all to God. This type of prayer has the ability to cast out fear, lessen worry and decrease stress. Prayer of this nature can provide a new outlook on problems and situations, with insights into forgiving others and receiving forgiveness for oneself.

In a prayer of petition, a personal plea is made to God. The therapeutic value of a prayer of petition is found throughout the ages. In this kind of prayer, the individual simply asks God to intervene and heal.

Wakefield describes Intercession as "prayer with, for and on behalf of another person, group of people or event of the world, which is undertaken by an individual or even the world." Church healing ministries and individual prayer warriors are actively engaged in this type of prayer for the sick and the spiritually distressed.

Prayer and its effects on healing

It is thought that prayer helps the body to heal, partially by triggering mechanisms for counteracting stress and promoting positive emotions thereby releasing the body's natural capacity for healing. Prayer has been shown to activate the immune, hormonal, and cardiovascular systems of the body leading to healing of disease, illness or injury. Prayer has been found to cause beneficial changes in the body, such as decreased heart rate, decreased blood pressure, and decreased episodes of angina in cardiology patients. Several studies have confirmed that there is an association between prayer and fewer hospitalizations and shorter hospital stays. In fact, a review of 1200 studies examining the relationship between prayer and health indicate that more than half of such studies show a significant positive connection.

In a 1988 study, a prayer group was instructed to pray for an experimental group with heart disease patients, while others in a control group were not prayed for. At the end of the study, the group that was prayed for had documented benefits. This group of patients required 20% less antibiotics than the unremembered group. They were two and a half times less likely to suffer congestive heart failure and the same group of patients was less likely to suffer cardiac arrest and had shorter hospitalizations.

The Duke University Studies

In the late 1990's, a series of studies on the effect of prayer and healing were conducted at Duke University. A 1997 study looked at the effects of spirituality on healing in older adults. Researchers found that those who attended religious services were less likely to have undesirably high levels of a protein called interleukin-6, resulting in a healthier immune system than those who didn't attend church. In a 1998 study of 4000 adults, researchers found that those who prayed daily and attended religious services weekly had 40% less hypertension than those who did not pray or attended service. In another study of 157 hospitalized adults with moderate to high levels of pain, prayer as an adjunct to pain medications was reported by 76% as the most common self-reported means of controlling pain (Koenig and Larson, 1998).

7 THE HEALING POWER OF PRAYER – PART 2

In last week's article, we talked about types of prayer and its effects on healing. This week we will review some recent scientific studies, many conducted by researchers who try to dispute its power. An article published in the April 2005 Journal of Science and Healing, titled "Are prayer experiments legitimate, twenty criticisms," looked closely at the idea that prayer can actually influence outcomes in a positive manner.

Often the effect of prayer is attributed to the placebo or Hawthorne effects. The Hawthorne effect is seen when attention is focused on a person; we tend to improve when we are being watched. A very interesting study by psychologist Bernard R. Grad, of McGill University disputed the placebo effect when he explored healing prayers on healing of surgical wounds and tumors in animals, and also the rate of growth of plants, finding prayer had positive effects in both instances. Experiments in nonhuman subjects are important because they eliminate the placebo effect, one of the most common objections lodged against prayer.

A 2016 study looked at the effect on the brain of healing prayers on depression and traumatic memories. Depression rooted in childhood trauma is very hard to treat. To document the effects of prayer in the brain, functional MRIs were performed prior to and after a 6-week prayer intervention. A functional MRI lights up different areas of the brain based on activity, and in depressed persons, specific areas of the brain are either depressed, or working overtime (obsessive thoughts). The functional MRI demonstrated increased activity in the front part of the brain during focus on the traumatic memory after the prayer intervention. Changes in activity in the left part of the brain correlated with improvement in depressive symptoms. Researchers concluded that the increased activity in the front part of the brain after healing prayer may be associated with having better control over emotions. Healing prayer may help to dissociate the memory of the trauma from feelings associated with it, an effect shown on the functional MRI.

A study published in Nov. 2005 looked at the efficacy of distant healing, also known as intercessory prayer, in clinical outcomes in patients with HIV-AIDS. 156 patients with a history of AIDS were assigned to 3 different groups: (1) 10 weeks of prayer/distant healing from professional healers, (2) 10 weeks of prayer/distant healing from nurses with no prior training or experience in distant healing, or, (3) no distant healing. Despite being blind to group assignment, subjects receiving intercessory prayers were significantly more likely to guess that they had been receiving healing than were subjects randomized to the no-treatment control group. In other words, they felt the prayers that were being sent to them. In this study, distant healing or prayer from a distance did not appear to improve selected clinical outcomes in the HIV patients studied.

How to Pray

Jesus answers this question in Matthew 6:5-13

"And when you pray, do not be like the hypocrites, for they love to pray standing in the synagogues and on the street corners to be seen by others. Truly I tell you, they have received their reward in full. But when you pray, go into your room, close the door and pray to your Father, who is unseen. Then your Father, who sees what is done in secret, will reward you. And when you pray, do not keep on babbling like pagans, for they think they will be heard because of their many words. Do not be like them, for your Father knows what you need before you ask him.

"This, then, is how you should pray:

"'Our Father which art in heaven,
hallowed be thy name,
thy kingdom come,
thy will be done,
on earth as it is in heaven.
Give us today our daily bread.
And forgive us our debts,
as we forgive our debtors.
And lead us not into temptation,
but deliver us from the evil: For
thine is the kingdom, and the
power, and the glory, for ever. Amen.

8 REVISITING TURMERIC

When I first wrote about turmeric a couple of years ago, it was in the process of making a comeback. Used mostly as an anti-inflammatory and for aches and pains, there are many more uses for turmeric, equally impressive as its pain-relieving properties. We will review some of the lesser-known uses for this essential herb. The medicinal part is the rhizome, or root, that looks similar to ginger root.

Anti-Obesity

Turmeric has many functions in the body, including anti-obesity. Contributing to obesity is leptin, a hormone produced by fat cells. Several replicated studies have shown that the concentration of leptin in the cell is significantly decreased by turmeric. In one study, rats were divided into four groups: a normal diet group, a high fat and high cholesterol group, and high fat and high cholesterol groups supplemented with turmeric in two different concentrations; 2.5% and 5%.

In the animals treated with turmeric, the levels of free fatty acids and leptin were decreased in a dose-dependent manner. Further studies of the treated animals showed that leptin helped to break down abdominal fat cells.

Inhaling Turmeric

Rarely used today, medicinal smoke has long been in the arsenal of man's natural remedies. It is common in some Asian countries to burn turmeric rhizomes to relieve nose and chest congestion. A 2016 study looked at the active components of ash smudges from burned turmeric. With smoke there are always nanoparticles, and turmeric smoke is no exception. The researchers found that smudges from turmeric smoke had both antimicrobial and anticancer properties. The researchers concluded that inhaling turmeric smoke might be one method of absorbing the medicinal properties of the herb.

Oral Health

Turmeric extracts have been shown to have destructive activity against bacteria in the mouth that can lead to cavities and other problems of the teeth and gums.

A 2016 study looked at using turmeric in homemade toothpaste powder to control *streptococcus mutans* in the mouth; the bacteria that causes cavities.

The dental powder was inspired from an ancient Indian powder, which is still being used in remote areas where modern toothpaste is not available. The four main constituents of the powder are alum, turmeric, cloves and salt all ground into a fine powder.

The dental powder showed effective antimicrobial activity against Streptococcus mutans in the laboratory setting.

Alzheimer's Treatment

It is generally though that Alzheimer's is due to amyloid, a type of protein plaque found in the brains of Alzheimer's Disease (AD) patients. Recent studies suggest that amyloid begins accumulating in the brain 10 – 20 years before the clinical onset of AD. If you can slow the build-up of amyloid, it is thought you can stave off Alzheimer's.

Turmeric binds both amyloid fibrils and helps to keep amyloid particles from clumping together and causing problems. The deposits of amyloid in the brains of affected patients are the pathological hallmarks of Alzheimer's disease (AD). When turmeric was administered to animal subjects, it effectively suppressed amyloid formation in the mouse brain.

Memory and Learning

A 2016 study looked at how long term use of turmeric extract can improve memory related learning in aged and Alzheimer disease subjects.

The results of the investigation revealed that turmeric extract provides beneficial effects on the learning ability of old rats and Alzheimer's disease model rats by providing anti-inflammatory action and protection of existing brain cells.

A very exciting finding shows that combining turmeric with the common Alzheimer drug Aricept (donepezil) improves learning and memory activity in human subjects.

The main concern about Turmeric is bioavailability, how much can be absorbed into the body. Other than occasional allergies, turmeric is very safe.

9 TYLENOL VS. ASPIRIN

When choosing over the counter pain relievers, there are essentially three choices, aspirin, Tylenol or ibuprofen.

Of the three, aspirin is the only natural product (with the ingredient salicin, found in willow bark), causing the fewest side effects. With a strong campaign by the makers of Tylenol proclaiming, "9 out of 10 Doctors prescribe Tylenol," and an over-hyped warning about Reye's syndrome due to aspirin, a lot of folks are missing its remarkable pain relieving properties.

Aspirin acts at the site of damaged tissue to block the start of the nerve signal to the brain, the mechanism by which we experience pain. It does this by blocking prostaglandins, the agents responsible for sensitizing nerve endings. In addition to causing pain, Prostaglandins are also responsible for inflammation, fever and the clotting of platelets in the blood.

On the other hand, it is not fully understood how Tylenol (acetaminophen) works. While Tylenol belongs to a class of painkillers known as non-opioid analgesics that also includes aspirin, ibuprofen, and prescription drugs such as Celebrex, Tylenol is different from aspirin in that it doesn't block pain in the peripheral nervous system, only the central nervous system.

Tylenol is a weak analgesic and has no anti-inflammatory properties. While it does reduce fever, it does so by a different mechanism than aspirin, and often fever goes up for a period after receiving Tylenol before it subsides. While Tylenol is ok for minor aches and pains, it won't reduce swelling or inflammation.

Reye's Syndrome and Aspirin's bad rap

Aspirin fell out of favor in the mid 1980's when it was thought to be associated with Reye's syndrome when given to children with viral illnesses, especially chicken pox. Reye's syndrome is a rare but serious condition that causes swelling in the liver and brain. It most often affects children and teenagers recovering from a viral infection, most commonly the flu or chickenpox, and presents with signs and symptoms such as confusion, seizures and loss of consciousness.

Around the time aspirin was thought to cause Reye's syndrome, Johnson & Johnson, the maker of Tylenol, was faced with a crisis. In late 1982, seven people died after taking Extra-Strength Tylenol capsules that were laced with cyanide. There was a nationwide panic, and Johnson and Johnson launched a very effective public relations campaign.

A few studies, now being disputed, linked the use of aspirin to the development of Reye's syndrome in children, leading the CDC, the U.S. Surgeon General, the American Academy of Pediatrics and the FDA to recommend that aspirin and combination products containing aspirin not be given to children under 19 years of age during episodes of fever-causing illnesses. Obviously this restriction resulted in a huge boost to the manufacturers of Tylenol.

Among the evidence emerging that aspirin doesn't cause Reye's syndrome is the fact that Kawasaki disease in children is treated with high doses of aspirin, but Reye's syndrome is very uncommon in these children, indicating it is time to rethink the link between aspirin and this illness. A 2004 study published in the Archive of Disease in Childhood relates that in Japan alone, up to 200 000 children have received Aspirin for Kawasaki disease. Interestingly, only one case of Reye syndrome associated with Kawasaki disease has ever been reported, and only in the Japanese literature.

The diagnosis of "Reye Syndrome" greatly decreased when genetic testing was becoming available. A study of 49 survivors of cases diagnosed as "Reye's Syndrome" showed that the majority of the surviving patients had various metabolic disorders that were actually responsible for the disease, not aspirin.

As the usage of aspirin decreases, there has been an increase in various allergic diseases, and some researchers feel this may be due in part to the decreased use of aspirin with its anti-inflammatory action that works to suppress allergic reactions.

Tylenol Toxicity

The main side effect of aspirin is bleeding, which can be closely monitored. In general, if you cut yourself, your blood should clot within 2 minutes. If your bleeding time is longer than that, you should likely cut back on your aspirin use – consulting with your health care provider, of course.

Tylenol comes with a whole set of problems. New research is showing that use of Tylenol while pregnant can lead to asthma in children. Tylenol is currently under increased scrutiny by the FDA due to the risk of intentional and unintentional overdose-related liver toxicity. Acetaminophen is responsible for an estimated 48% of all acute liver failure diagnoses. People with liver problems should never take Tylenol in my opinion. We recently lost a member of our community to liver cirrhosis (in a person who never drank) that was linked to Tylenol use for headaches.

Rethink aspirin for your aches and pains. It is the cheapest drug out there, helps to prevent stroke and heart attack, and a truly natural product.

10 BUTTERNUT

In Missouri, we are blessed to still have some Butternut trees (Juglans cinerea). A species of walnut, it is also referred to as white walnut. Lumber from the butternut tree is very valuable in making fine furniture, as it carves easily and glues together well. The tree is native to eastern North America, ranging from Canada down through Missouri and Arkansas.

Butternut trees are in trouble in Missouri due to susceptibility to cankers, but not yet endangered. George O. White Nursery here is Licking is actively seeking seeds from this special tree, with hopes of growing them into seedlings that can be distributed and planted all over the state. If you are fortunate enough to have some butternut seeds, they are best sown as soon as it they are ripe in individual deep pots in a cold frame. The seed (nut) usually germinates in late winter or the spring. Plant the seedlings in early summer and protect from winter cold until they get established. You can also store the seed in the refrigerator over the winter, and then sow in the early spring.

Butternut trees are medium sized, and can grow 40-60 feet tall. The green leaves are opposite on the branches with serrated edges. Butternut bark is light gray. While walnuts are round, the nut from the butternut is longer than it is wide with deep ridges, and has a green husk like the walnut.

Use as a food

Butternuts are rich in flavor, similar to the walnuts with which we are familiar, although the fruit is smaller. Like many trees one wouldn't normally consider tapping, the sap from the butternut tree can be tapped and used as a sweet drink, or boiled down to make syrup. The nuts can be eaten raw, or ground into a powder that can be added to soup, stews, or used for flour. The nuts can also be used to press into edible oil.

Medicinal Uses

Most of the medicinal properties are found in the inner bark of the roots, best collected in May or June.

Moerman discussed the use Native American use of butternut. The Cherokee made pills from the bark to treat toothaches. The Iroquois used nut oil from the butternut to condition hair, an infusion of the bark to induce labor in pregnant women, and applied the bark to wounds. The nut oil was also mixed with bear grease to use as a mosquito repellant.

Modern herbalists recommend butternut as a gentle laxative, and oil pressed from the nut is said to remove tapeworms. Rubbing the skin with the bark brings blood to the surface, thought to relieve the pain of arthritis and rheumatism by improving circulation to the affected area. There are also reports of Butternut lowering cholesterol levels and promoting the clearance of waste products and toxins by the liver.

Antibiotic activity

In a 2000 study, bark extract from butternut was found to be active against MRSA and other forms of bacteria, yeast and fungus The study also demonstrated a correlation between frequency of traditional medicinal use by Native Americans and antimicrobial activity of extracts indicating that the traditional knowledge "encompasses an understanding of aspects of chemical ecology."

In a 2003 study, several plant extracts, but especially those from ginger and butternut had pronounced antifungal activity against a wide variety of fungi, including strains that were highly resistant to strong anti-fungal medications like amphotericin B and ketoconazole.

Other Uses

Butternut can be used to make a yellow brown dye that is extracted from the bark by boiling. Using a chemical containing iron to increase adherence of the dye to the fabric changes butternut dye to a gray color, and was used during the Civil War to dye the Confederate uniforms, hence the name "butternuts."

Precautions

Butternut appears to be safe in any form, although shouldn't be used by pregnant women as it may induce labor.

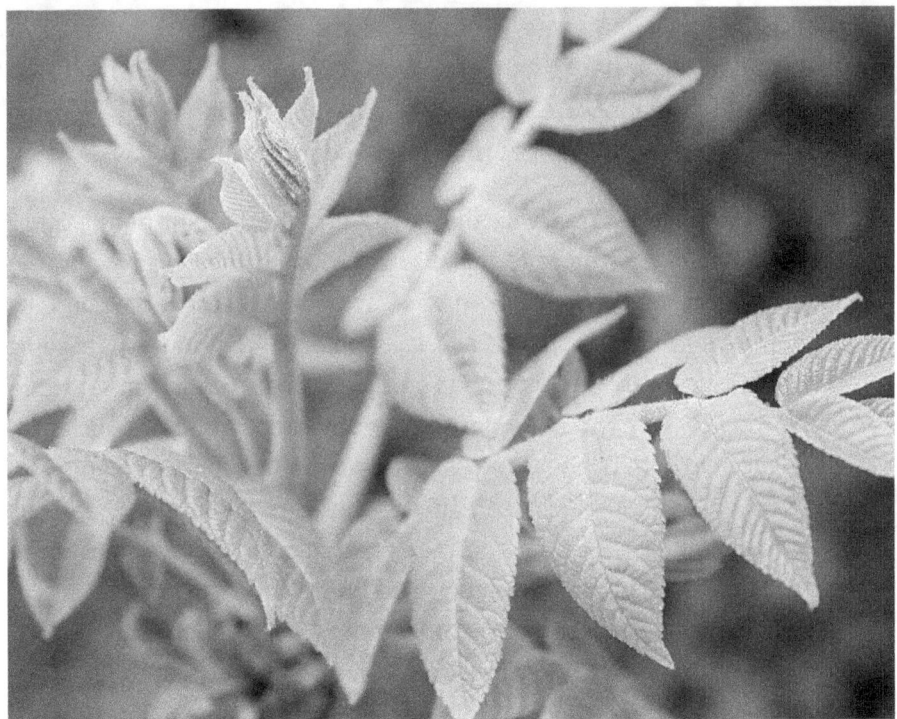

Butternut has green leaves with serrated edges that are opposite on the branches. (Photo courtesy mdc.mo.gov)

11 FLU SHOT? NO THANK YOU

It was 1977, and the Swine flu was in the news, being compared to the Spanish Flu pandemic. With a $137 million dollar campaign to immunize every man, woman and child, and vaccine manufacturers held immune from lawsuits, the vaccine caused many more problems than the disease it was supposed to prevent. Ad hoc analysis shows that the swine flu was confined to Fort Dix, and posed no threat to the general public. Only one person, an Army recruit, died from the flu outbreak.

3 people died immediately after receiving the vaccine. Thousands of others became intensely ill with flu symptoms. Five hundred others contracted Guillain-Barré after receiving the shot, and at least 25 of them died. I am one of the survivors of the swine flu vaccine. I contracted Guillain-Barré after receiving the shot in my nursing program, strongly encouraged, but not mandatory as it is today.

About a week after receiving the flu shot, my legs went numb, and I couldn't urinate. My mom took me to the ER, and they gave me a pain shot and sent me home. I saw my family doctor the next day, and my bladder was ready to rupture, as I still couldn't urinate. Despite being numb, my legs were exquisitely painful with any touch. I was sent to a major medical center, and underwent dozens of painful tests, including a lumbar myelogram where they inject dye into your spinal column and put you on a tilt table to spread the dye throughout your nervous system while taking x-rays. When the tests came back, I was diagnosed with Guillain-Barré, a paralyzing neuromuscular disorder. I was fortunate, as my paralysis only extended to my waist, and after a month in the hospital I eventually recovered. Others weren't so lucky. In some cases the paralysis extended upward to the chest and even neck level, making it impossible for the victim to breathe, requiring mechanical ventilation. Those that recovered from this bear the mark of the disease, a telltale tracheotomy scar on their neck.

My parents had to pay my extensive medical bills back then, as it took awhile for the reality of the Swine Flu Vaccine causing unprecedented cases of Guillain-Barré to become evident. When folks started to sue vaccine makers, Congress granted them total immunity from civil litigation due to injuries or deaths resulting from their product, instead of requiring the drug companies to produce safer vaccines.

Vaccine victims today have to file for compensation though the National Vaccine Injury Compensation Program that was established by Congress and paid for with your tax dollars. In 2016, 44428 cases were posted of vaccine injuries, ranging from prolonged pain at injection site, to seizures, neurological disorders and death. In the first 2 weeks of 2017, 364 cases were already filed.

Help Yourself

Influenza A is the strain most likely to cause a pandemic, and results released this week from the Texas county health depart show that Influenza A cases outnumber those of the B variety by a ratio of 130 to 50. Many of those testing positive were previously vaccinated for the flu, with one health provider reporting that of the last 10 cases they tested, 100% had been vaccinated. This is not uncommon. A review of the literature shows that often the CDC comes back and states the millions of flu shots administered were a mismatch to the specific virus.

There are readily available natural methods to keep us healthy through flu season. Don't forget to spend at least 10 – 15 minutes a day in the sunlight. Most flu cases occur between Oct. and March, when we get the least amount of sunshine – an important element that helps our body produce Vitamin D, essential for a strong immune system.

Pine extract preparations, both from the needles and cones, have been proven to be effective against Influenza A. A 2010 study looked at the virus inhibiting activity of pine needle extract against 2 highly contagious strains of Avian influenza Virus A, and found the extract decreased the amount of virus present in cells by up to 50%.

Another study evaluated the use of pinecone extract (PCE) against the influenza virus. PCE appears to target RNA synthesis in the virus itself, preventing it from multiplying.

Disinfectant

Pine extracts are effective against a wide range of bacteria, fungus and viruses. We all remember Pine-Sol, but you have to make your own, as the commercial version no longer contains pine extract, only alcohols. Makers of the new product cite lack of supply and expense as the reason pine oil is no longer a part of their product.

12 CHARCOAL

By Tamara Glascock

Charcoal seems to be the trendy new health product, but the benefits of activated charcoal have been known for millennium. Hippocrates (460-370 B.C.) and the ancient Egyptians employed the use of charcoal for a variety of ailments. Most notably for its ability to rid the body of toxins and impurities.

Activated charcoal is made using coconut shells or select types of wood. Coconut shells are the preferred option due to its renewability, and because charcoal made from wood has the potential to cause an allergic reaction in those with sensitivity to certain types of nuts and woods. The charcoal is created through a process of steam, heat and washing. The result is a substance that can adsorb up to 350 times its weight in gases, liquids and toxins.

That is *adsorb*, not absorb. The difference? When something is absorbed it is taken in and disappears, as with a sponge. When something is *adsorbed* it works like a magnet, drawing substances to its surface and holding onto them tightly.

Charcoal's uniqueness lies in the range of substances that it is capable of adsorbing. It has been shown to adsorb toxic gases and chemicals, especially those from prescription drugs, venom, poison, and toxic metals, making it exceptionally valuable in helping cleanse the system from drug addiction, and helping those with intestinal issues like excessive gas, diarrhea, heartburn and ulcers. It is commonly found in emergency rooms around the world, and is an absolute must-have for every home medicine cabinet.

The newest trend for activated charcoal is in the beauty arena. Little wonder, since the benefits of charcoal are often seen after a single use. Charcoal draws impurities from the skin, whitens teeth, freshens breath, and reduces blackheads and acne.

When purchasing activated charcoal, look for a source that specifies what the charcoal is derived from. Always choose organic, as this ensures it is free from chemical processing which can cause many adverse reactions.

Charcoal is available in three forms: tablets, capsules and powder. Tablets should be crushed or chewed before swallowing, and are the least effective. Capsules take time to break down in the digestive system, requiring more of them to get the desired results. The powder is least expensive, most versatile, and most effective way to use charcoal.

A word of caution; it is not selective in the substances it adsorbs. This means that it pulls out the good with the bad. Vitamins, nutrients, amino acids and digestive enzymes are pulled from the body. Charcoal should not be taken long-term.

In the home, setting a small bowl in your fridge or pantry will eliminate odors.

If your goal is to detox the body, or to help control gas and bloating, take 1 teaspoon twice daily on an empty stomach. Be sure to drink at least 100 ounces of water per day while taking charcoal.

To whiten teeth and help eliminate tooth or gum issues, use charcoal twice a week in place of your normal toothpaste. Dip your toothbrush in the powder. Brush your teeth as usual, allowing the charcoal to remain on the teeth for 3-5 minutes. Rinse until the water is clear.

For bites and stings, mix charcoal powder and ground flax seed with enough boiling water to create a semi-thick paste. Apply the paste, extending it out past the affected area. Cover the paste with plastic.

Cover the plastic with a natural-fiber cloth like cotton or wool. Secure it with an ace bandage and leave on 8-10 hours. Wash with lukewarm salt water after removing the poultice. Repeat daily until the area has healed.

Editor's Note: Tamara Glascock is a local herbalist and natural medicine practitioner who lives in Edgar Springs.

11 TIME TO HARVEST YOUR BANDAGES

We are all familiar with the tall, yellow-flowered shoots of the common mullein plant, *Verbascum thapsus.* Verbascum is derived from Latin word meaning barbascum barba or beard, referring to the beardlike filaments. The word mullein comes from the Latin word mollis, or soft. Before attaining heights of up to 5 feet, the plant starts out in a basal rosette stage. The silver-green leaves are wonderfully soft to the touch, and have an added benefit of being a hemostat (bleeding stopper) with antimicrobial properties.

Mullein is a truly medicinal plant with a long history of successful use in treating respiratory infections and chronic cough. The dried leaves are sold online, and can actually be smoked to treat stubborn breathing problems. This use has a valid basis: bacteria known to cause respiratory infection are sensitive to mullein, especially Klebsiella pneumonia and staph aureus. Mullein treatment has been scientifically proven today, and somehow our forebears discovered it by trial and error. The people of Rome and Ireland called mullein "lungwort" because it was used to treat lung disease in both humans and livestock.

As the medicinal uses of mullein were discussed in a previous article, this week's focus will be on the uses of the leaves in treating cuts and inflamed tissues. The leaves are best harvested in the first year of the plant's growth when there appears only a rosette of large, thick leaves, approximately 6 inches long, with a soft, dense mass of hairs on both sides. These soft, fuzzy leaves are so absorbent there are reports of them being worn in the shoes to keep feet dry and warm.

The fuzzy leaves absorb blood and help it to clot. They also have antibacterial action against Staphlococcus, and are safe to apply to open wounds. When used to treat an infected, draining wound, the whole leaf should be applied moist, soaking it in a weak salt solution if necessary. Allow the leaf to dry, at least twelve hours. When you peel the leaf off, the tiny tendrils will adhere to the dead tissue, debriding the wound and leaving only the healthy tissue behind. Several studies have shown that the use of mullein decreases scar formation. In several studies, topical application of herbal extract of mullein was associated the deposit of new tissue, with a 20% boost to tissue healing.

In addition to being antiseptic and stopping bleeding, mullein leaves are also anti-inflammatory, helping to decrease the pain and swelling in injured tissues. The flowers of mullein also have pain-relieving properties in addition to being anti-inflammatory. For hemorrhoids, application of a moistened mullein leaf works much like an over the counter preparation to relieve pain and shrink swollen tissues.

Mullein flower oil is well known as a gentle, effective earache remedy, and this oil can also be used topically on any inflammation or nerve pain. Earache drops made from mullein also have strong bactericidal properties.

Nutrition

Mullein is fully edible, and is an important source of vitamins, minerals, and health-promoting fatty acids.

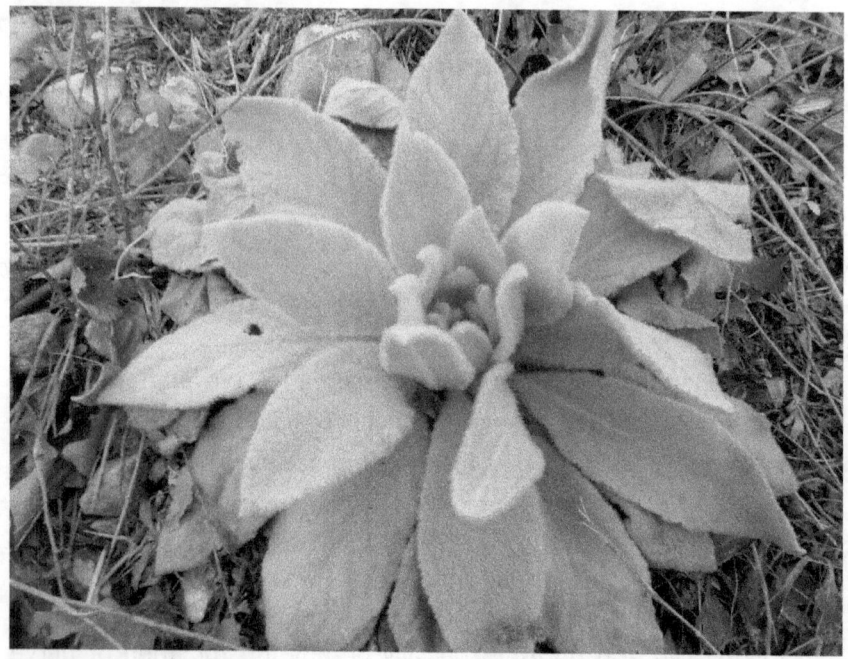

Mullein plants like stony ground in woodland clearings, and also grow along roadsides like this plant spotted along Kimble Rd. in Licking.

14 ALL AROUND THE MULBERRY BUSH

The fruit of the Mulberry tree is a delicious ingredient in home-made jam, but the native Ozark red mulberry tree *Morus Rubra* offers much more than a tasty treat. The roots, bark and leaves have antioxidant, antiviral, antibacterial, anti-inflammatory, cholesterol lowering, blood sugar regulation and neuro protective qualities. The leaves are popular in Korea and Japan for diabetic patients and are also used as nutritional supplements.

In addition to the native American red mulberry, there are over 150 species of Mulberry trees worldwide, and most familiar to Ozarkians is the white mulberry *Morus Alba*, an introduced plant from Asia, used for silkworm cultivation. Mulberry trees are very strong and adaptable, resistant to drought, and stable below 0 degrees centigrade. Our native red mulberry can live up to 75 years. White mulberry is named for the color of its flowers, not its fruit, that can be either red or black. White mulberry is considered an escaped invasive, and is found in urban areas. The native red mulberry is found in natural settings, scattered throughout the forest. Even if you don't want to reap the health benefits of mulberry, having a tree on your place will protect other fruit trees from birds and squirrels, as they greater prefer mulberries over any other fruit!

Nutrition

The different species of Mulberry offer significant nutritional benefits in varying amounts. Our native Red Mulberry is highest in protein with 2 grams of protein. At just 60 calories per cup, it also contains 2 grams of fiber, and 85% of the RDA for Vitamin C and 14% for Iron.

Atherosclerosis

A 2010 study examined the effect of a water extract of the leaves from the Red Mulberry plant on atherosclerosis (hardening of the arteries with plaque). Treatment with the extract for just 5 consecutive days showed significant improvement in body weight and blood cholesterol levels. Factors adversely affecting the lining of blood vessels were reversed to near normal. The researchers concluded "our study shows that aqueous leaf extract of *Morus rubra*, (400 mg/g) significantly improves glucose and fat metabolism and possesses significant anti-atherosclerotic activity."

Obesity

What I find the most exciting is the effect of Mulberry leaf extract on obesity. A 2014 study looked at the effect of mulberry leaf extract on fat cells. They found that without any apparent toxic effects, mulberry leaf extract prevented fat accumulation in the cells, concluding it is has potential as an anti-obesity drug, with no side effects.

The fruit of the mulberry also aids in weight loss. A study published in February of this year examined the effect of mulberry juice on brown fat. Brown fat generates body heat by burning calories – resulting in weight loss. Infants have very high levels of brown fat, which is why they don't shiver when it's cold. We tend to lose brown fat as we age, and it is largely absent in obese people. Mulberry juice supports the production of beneficial brown fat.

A 2013 study found that mulberry juice prevents diet-induced obesity through increases in adiponectin, a protein hormone that regulates glucose regulation and fat metabolism. Higher levels of adiponectin are seen with lower body fat percentages, and are elevated in patients with anorexia nervosa.

Blood sugar stabilization

A study from January of this year looked at the effect of mulberry tea in the reduction of abnormally high postprandial (after-eating) blood glucose levels in Type 2 diabetic patients.

Fasting blood sugar levels were recorded, then after the consumption of plain tea or mulberry tea, post-meal blood glucose levels were measured, showing a highly significant decrease in the glucose level in response to mulberry tea in all the test patients compared with the subjects that drank plain tea. The effect on blood sugar level was also found to be very large.

In a 2010 animal study, red mulberry leaf extract was orally administered to diabetic rats daily for 21 days. Blood samples were drawn to measure glucose tolerance and lipid parameters. The extract showed a dose-dependent fall in fasting blood glucose with an increase in plasma insulin levels. Examination of pancreatic tissue revealed an increased number of islets and beta-cells in extract-treated diabetic rats. This is extremely important, because these cells are where insulin is produced, and they are either absent or decreased in diabetic patients.

Oral Health

The mulberry fruit itself has excellent anti-microbial activity against many forms of bacteria, yeasts, and fungi, including the common oral pathogen that causes cavities - Streptococcus mutans. A few studies have studied the used of red mulberry juice in oral health, and it was found to be an excellent "temporary storage medium for the maintenance of periodontal ligament cell viability in avulsed teeth." In other words, if your tooth is knocked out, save it in red mulberry juice until you get to the dentist and it can likely be re-implanted.

Marie Lasater

15 CREEPING CHARLIE

Creeping Charlie, Latin name *Glechoma hederacea*, grows throughout Missouri. Not really a native, it was introduced to North America from Europe and is now considered naturalized. Creeping Charlie has kidney shaped leaves with scalloped edges. Like other members of the mint family, the stem is square. The plant flowers in the spring in clusters of two to three flowers with blue or lavender petals. Creeping Charlie grows well in the woods, but can take over lawns, forming large patches as it spreads by rhizome (underground roots) in addition to seeds. Not everyone is a fan of Creeping Charlie! Invasive or not, bees love this plant, and will benefit if you leave it in your lawn, a fairly easy thing to do because it can't be eradicated with mowing.

Use as a food

Creeping Charlie was deliberately imported to the United States by early European settlers because it was so useful, both as a nutritional food source with the added benefit of medicinal properties. Besides its obvious use as a salad green, in years past, Creeping Charlie has been used to clarify beer, and as a vegetarian substitute for rennet in cheese-making. High in vitamin C, and available during the winter months, Creeping Charlie can be made into a nutritious tea, especially important to those who may not have access to citrus fruit. Creeping Charlie is also high in potassium.

Medicinal Uses

Creeping Charlie has been used in traditional medicine to treat several illnesses, ranging from asthma to diabetes. It is an anti-inflammatory and has anti-oxidant activity. The English herbalist John Gerard recommended the plant in the treatment of tinnitus – ringing in the ears. When used to treat tinnitus, it can be consumed as a tea, or a drop of essential oil made from the plant can be instilled directly on the eardrum.

High Blood Pressure

The effect of an extract of Creeping Charlie on high blood pressure was tested in a 2007 study with laboratory animals. Animals fed a diet containing the extract for 14-28 days had a significantly lowered blood pressure. It was theorized that blood pressure was lowered due to a higher excretion of sodium.

Diabetes

In a study published in 2004, an extract of Creeping Charlie was added to the diet of diabetic lab animals once a day for 6 days. Results showed that the plant extract had an anti-diabetic effect.

Skin Whitening

Melanin is a pigment in the upper layer of your skin that gives it color. Sometimes melanin is in overdrive, and is accelerated by ultraviolet light. The good aspect of extra melanin production is the fact it can create a tan that helps protect deeper layers of skin from UV rays, but sometimes too much melanin can cause unsightly liver (age) spots. Several studies have shown that Creeping Charlie inhibits melanin, and is an effective component of whitening cosmetics in the form of lotions and creams used to treat age spots.

Safety

In humans, Creeping Charlie has a good safety profile, but according to Penn Veterinary Medicine, horses are susceptible to some of the oils contained in the plant. Symptoms include excess salivation and sweating, dilated pupils and even pulmonary edema. Dogs and other animals are not affected, but horses should not be allowed to graze in areas where the plant is present.

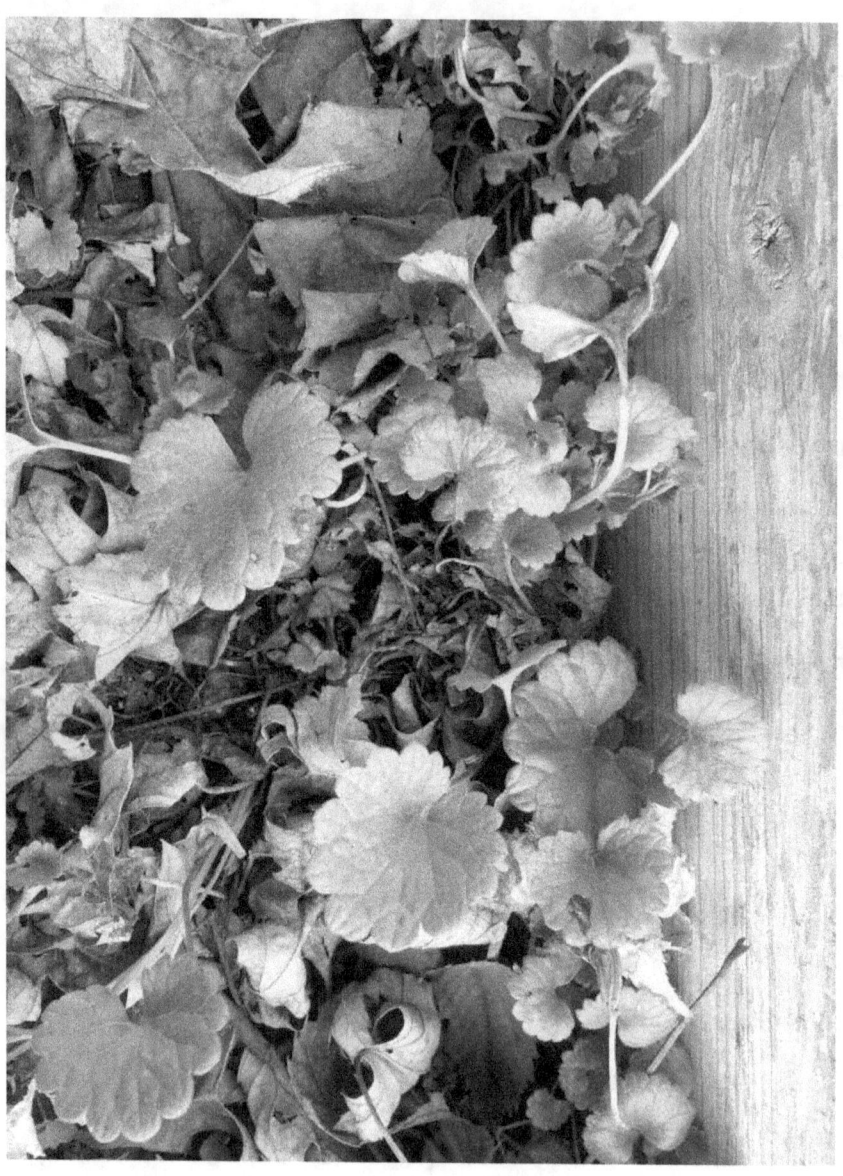

Creeping Charlie has kidney shaped leaves with scalloped edges.

16 MALLOW

Oh, what a salad you can find in front of the Licking Post office! Never noticed previously, there are luscious patches of common mallow, one of those delightful plants that are both nutritious and have medical uses.

In the same family as okra (Malvaceae), all parts of the plant are edible, and the fruit of the plant can be substituted for capers. The young mallow leaves can be used fresh in salads and substituted for lettuce, while older leaves are better served cooked. Flower petals from the mallow are also popular in salads. The plant grows close to the ground and produces flowers that bloom from June to late autumn.

As discovered centuries ago, boiling the leaves releases a slimy substance, similar to that found in okra that can be used as a thickener for soups and stews and can be beaten like eggs to make a type of meringue. Mallow roots also release thick mucus when boiled. A tea can be made from the dried leaves. The plant is rich in Vitamins A and C, in addition to several minerals including calcium, magnesium, potassium, iron and selenium.

Yes, marshmallows do grow on trees - or actually inside the mallow plant. Ancient Egyptians made marshmallows by extracting the goo from a mallow plant and mixing it with nuts and honey. By the 1800's, candy makers in France were mixing the sap with egg whites and sugar, creating the product we know today. In mass manufacturing, mallow sap has been replaced with gelatin.

Medicinal Uses

Over 1000 plants in the malvaceae family contain healing mucilage. The native plant is used in natural medicine as an anti-inflammatory, a soothing film (demulcent), a moisturizer, diuretic, an expectorant and as a laxative.

Wound treatment

As a treatment for wounds, a tea is made with the slimy material found within the mallow stem in the aerial parts (those above the ground), steeped for 15 minutes in 1 cup of hot water.

Sore throat

A solution made from the healing mucilage in the plant can also be used as a gargle for sore throat and to soothe a persistent cough. Mallow gargle also reduces gum irritation; in addition to its moistening properties, it can reduce harmful oral bacteria.

Antibacterial

Extract from the mallow plant has been found effective against both gram negative and gram-positive bacteria and some forms of mycobacterium, a type of bacteria that includes tuberculosis. Mallow has also been reputed to prevent ulcers, perhaps by inhibiting *h.pylori*, the bacteria responsible for stomach ulcers.

Anti-inflammatory

Mallow extracts have high cox-1 inhibiting activity, similar to many anti-arthritis drugs. In a 2010 study that reviewed 1000 plants reported to anti-inflammatory activity, only nine demonstrated significant clinical evidence of therapeutic effect, with mallow being one of them. A compound called beta-sitosterol has been found in marshmallow, used to treat high cholesterol and trouble urinating due to an enlarged prostate. Taking beta-sitosterol significantly lowers total and bad (LDL) cholesterol levels, but doesn't raise good (HDL) cholesterol. .

Kidney problems

In traditional medicine, mallow is used to treat kidney and gallstones, and promote diuresis.

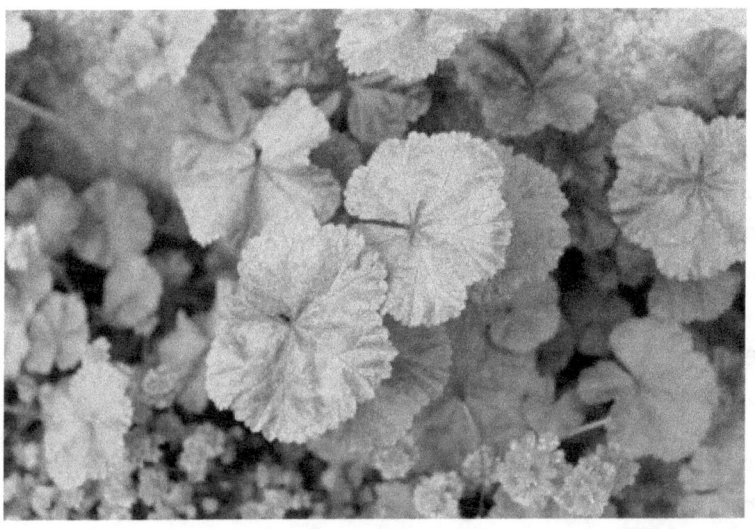

A lovely mallow plant, growing in front of the Licking Post Office.

17 KEFIR

Recently I received a bottle of home-processed kefir from a friend here in Licking. If you've never heard of kefir, it is a fermented product made from grains that comprise a specific and complex mixture of bacteria and yeasts. The nutritional composition of kefir varies according to the milk composition, the microbiological composition of the grains used, the time/temperature of fermentation and storage conditions. The microorganisms found in kefir have pro-biotic potential. They are able to adhere to the intestine, and interfere with problem bacteria, contributing to gut health.

Originally from Tibet and that region, kefir is becoming very popular locally due to its many positive health effects, including improved digestion and lactose tolerance, effect on cholesterol, antibacterial action, control of blood sugar, effect on blood pressure, anti-inflammatory effects, ability to fight cancer, and allergy reducing effects, to name a few. In fact, the name kefir means "well-being."

Kefir can easily and safely be made at home. There are many variations, and kefir can be ingested immediately after grain separation, or refrigerated to consume later. Starter cultures are available, but the final product has a lower number and variety of microorganisms than fermented milk produced from kefir grains.

Nutritional Analysis

Kefir grains look like cauliflower, and include 4.4% fat, 12.1% ash, 34.3% protein, vitamins B and K, tryptophan, calcium, phosphorus and magnesium.

Health Effects

Kefir can prevent several gastrointestinal disorders. Many people suffer from lactose intolerance. For milk products to be absorbed in the intestine, it has to be broken down by a specific enzyme, naturally present in kefir grains. Kefir has been shown to reduce to severity of flatulence (gas) due to milk products by up to 71%.

Antimicrobial properties

Consumption of kefir has a positive effect on life expectancy, thought to be due to competition between lactic acid bacteria found in the product and harmful bacteria, fungi, and yeasts. In essence, kefir robs these harmful organisms of nutrients they need to survive in the body.

Effect on Cholesterol

Pro-biotic dairy products such as kefir have been studied as one way to reduce cholesterol levels. In one analysis that included 13 studies with a total of 485 subjects, kefir and other pro-biotic dairy products were found to lower cholesterol by 6 – 40 mg/dl. It works by binding cholesterol in the intestine. In the laboratory setting, kefir was able to absorb 28 – 65% of cholesterol.

Control of Blood Sugar

Consuming kefir regularly has been shown to improve blood sugar levels. It is thought to decrease oxidative stress that raises blood sugar, and also to restore function of insulin receptors.

Effect on Blood Pressure

Kefir is able to inhibit the activity of an enzyme that raises blood pressure. Beneficial effects on blood pressure include blocking constriction of blood vessels and decreasing the level of sodium in the blood.

Cancer Prevention

In addition to clearing cholesterol, all bacterial strains isolated from kefir have the ability to bind to mutagens, which can then be excreted from the body, especially effective against colon cancer cells.

Other healing effects

Kefir has beneficial effects far beyond the intestine. Wounds, including burns, heal more quickly. Skin problems and atopic dermatitis improve when kefir is added to the diet.

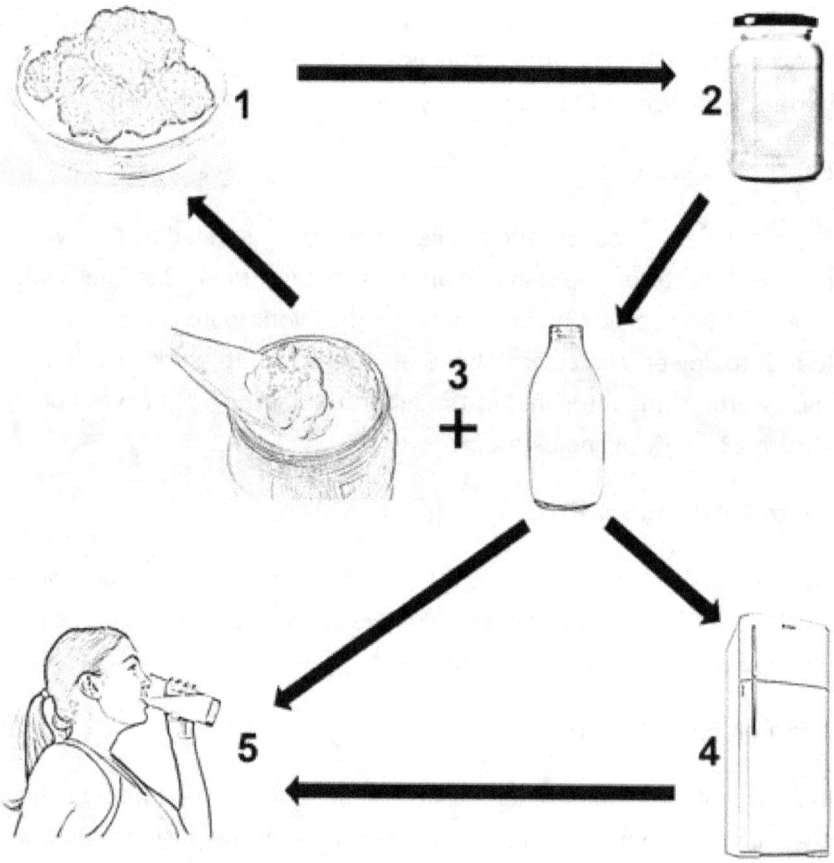

Home-made kefir. (1) Separation of kefir grains. (2) Addition of milk to the kefir grains in a half-open container at room temperature to ferment for 10 to 24 h. (3) Filtration and separation of kefir grains. Possible addition of the kefir grains to fresh milk to start a new fermentation. The kefir is adequate for consumption. (4) The kefir can be refrigerated (39°F). (5) The kefir is safe and ready to drink. Reproduced by Permission: Cambridge University Press.

18 GOATS RUE – IT'S WHERE METFORMIN COMES FROM

I firmly believe every helpful pharmaceutical product has a counterpart in nature. Supporting my theory, the popular drug for diabetes, Metformin, has its origin in Galega officinalis, commonly known as French lilac or Goat's Rue.

Goat's Rue is native to the Middle East, but grows easily in Missouri. In 1891, it was introduced into Utah as a forage crop, but escaped cultivation (How I love that term!) and wound up on the Federal noxious weed list. It is a helpful plant for bees, but as a forage plant, has proven toxic to livestock, which is where the name Goat's Rue originated. Rue, of course, means regret, and the plant has been shown to cause pulmonary edema, low blood pressure, paralysis and death in certain animals that consume too much of the plant. Despite these terrible symptoms, there are several suppliers of Goat's Rue online, where it is mainly sold to increase milk production in the breastfeeding mother, and also as a natural method to treat diabetes in dogs.

Prior to pharmaceutical manufacture, dried leaves of goat's rue were used as a treatment for diabetes. Dating back to medieval times, a tea made with Goat's Rue was used to treat frequent urination and bad breath with a sweet odor, now known as common diabetes symptoms. Researchers have found that the plant contains a substance called guanidine that has been shown to reduce blood sugar. In fact, the active ingredient in Goat's Rue is guanidine. In the 1920's and 1930's, a less toxic component of the plant was discovered, called galegine, also found naturally in Goat's Rue.

Metformin is helpful in type 2 diabetes, the type that doesn't require insulin. The guanidine found in Goat's Rue was discovered in 1922, and was found to have the most powerful sugar-lowering ingredient known at that time when tested in animals. When insulin took over for the treatment of diabetes, metformin was essentially forgotten until the 1940's and 50's. At that time, metformin was also found to have antiviral properties, and was used to treat influenza.

In 1957, a French physician studied galegine, isolated from Goat's Rue, and was the first to try in on diabetic humans. He named the new drug Glucophage (glucose eater.) The new drug became available in Europe in 1958, but it wasn't approved by the FDA for Type 2 Diabetes in the United States until 1994, and first marketing in early 1995. Today, nearly 120 million prescriptions are filled each year throughout the world.

Role in Treating Cancer

The ability of galegine to lower circulating insulin may be particularly important for the treatment of cancers known to be associated with high insulin levels, such as those of the breast and colon. It is thought to also directly inhibit cancer cells.

Galegine blocks the formation of glucose in the liver and helps carry glucose into the muscle tissue where it is used for energy. It enhances sensitivity to insulin, all effects that help to lower blood glucose.

Gelegine, in the form of metformin, was first found to protect against cancer in studies of diabetic patients. There were many reports of decreased cancer illness and deaths from cancer in diabetics taking standard doses of metformin.

While the majority of evidence supporting a role for metformin in the treatment of cancer has been derived from retrospective studies involving diabetics, some prospective clinical trials have been completed in non-diabetic patients. In a recent study, low doses of metformin (250 mg/day) reduced the number of precancerous lesions for colorectal in non-diabetic patients

Recent studies have demonstrated that metformin may also target cancer-initiating cells. For example, metformin inhibited the growth of a subpopulation of breast cancer cells shown to have such properties, and reduced their ability to form tumors in mice.

Other Uses

In addition to its use in diabetics, metformin is also effective in the treatment of polycystic ovarian syndrome.

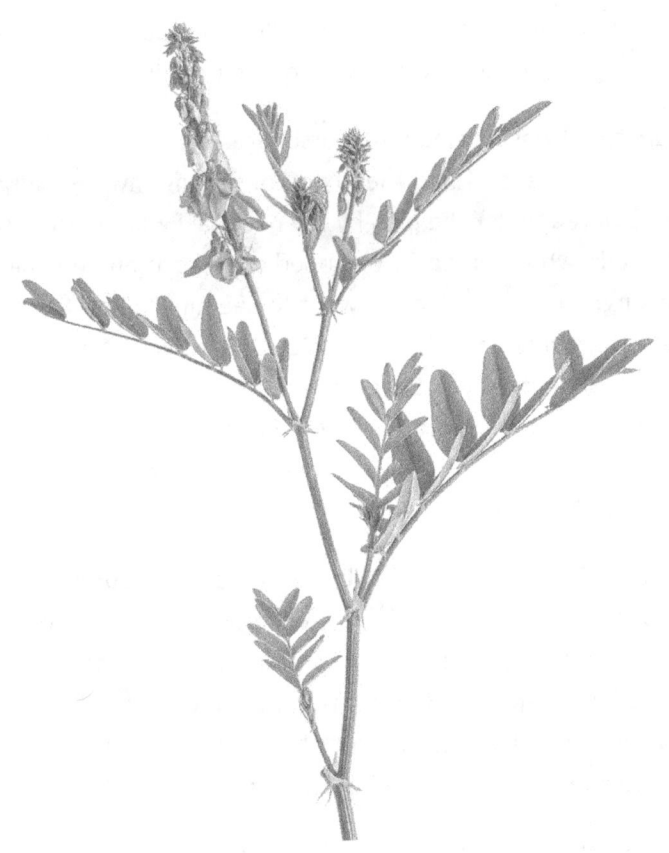

Goat's Rue contains the major active ingredient used in Metformin.

19 THE HIGH COST OF HEALTH INSURANCE
Is there a better way?

Last week I had a crown re-cemented. When I had the procedure performed 2 years ago, at a time when I had dental insurance, it cost $87. This time, because I was paying cash, the cost was only $52. Since insurance did not pay the full cost, I actually came out BEHIND having insurance, taking in account the high cost of the premiums.

Several years ago, I was bucked off a horse, breaking my shoulder. I was uninsured at the time, so I had the luxury of picking my own surgeon, not the one covered under the plan by the hospital I worked for. I called upon my friends who worked in orthopedics to recommend the best orthopedic surgeon. They did, and I went to see him. When I explained my situation, he agreed to perform a $12,000 surgery for $600. The difference was that it would be performed in an outpatient surgery center, and instead of recuperating in the hospital, I would have to go straight home and take care of myself. I healed perfectly, and was very glad I didn't have health insurance!

I don't think all insurance is bad. Obviously we need auto and home insurance, but these companies have to compete with each other for your business, and if you are dissatisfied with one, you can fire them and pick another company. Health insurance doesn't work that way. With managed care networks, they dictate which provider you can see, limiting choice and completely eliminating competition.

I've been a member of a health care sharing ministry for several years now. My "premiums," called shares, are sent directly to the person who has the medical expense, along with a note and a prayer. This works beautifully with no insurance company involved. There are no deductibles, but medical expense can't be submitted unless it exceeds $300.00.

Another issue with health insurance is the fact that your premiums may pay for things you do not want or need. At 60 years old, I don't need pregnancy coverage. In 1940, less than 10 percent of the population had health insurance, and just paid as they went on health care costs. It is clear that health insurance is inflationary.

One reason for having insurance is for a catastrophic expense. One way to cover this partially is by increasing your automobile policy to maximum medical coverage at a reasonable cost. Yes, there is a chance you may need expensive surgery or cancer therapy, but like putting $100 on black in the casino, the odds are against you on cashing in on your insurance investment. And too often, insurance finds a way not to pay for these catastrophic expenses, citing that the care was unnecessary or experimental.

Most folks I know without health insurance try to live a very healthy lifestyle, and try alternative and natural treatments first. They also know to ask their doctor to prescribe medications from the $4.00 list available at most pharmacies, if possible, and avoid the latest exorbitantly priced pharmaceutical.

One should always plan ahead for unexpected medical care. There are online services such as medibid.com and Surgery Center of Oklahoma that give you an upfront price quote for surgery and procedures; bringing competition to the marketplace.

Know your levels of care. The emergency room is a very expensive place to receive medical care, and your doctor's office or an urgent care clinic will treat you promptly, and cost a lot less. Everyone needs a primary care provider, a doctor or nurse practitioner who knows you, is willing to take cash as payment. I have one, and she is great.

20 HOME-BASED HELP FOR
ASTHMA SUFFERERS

Asthma can be a life-threatening illness, and folks who suffer with this ailment should be under the supervision of a health care provider. Those with severe asthma should never be without an inhaler nearby.

In years gone by, a rescue inhaler called Primatene Mist was available over the counter, but was banned in 2011. Primatene's main ingredient was epinephrine, used world wide to treat tracheal spasm. The inhaler wasn't banned due to the effective medication it contained, however, but was removed from the market to comply with the Montreal Protocol on Substances that Deplete the Ozone Layer. Prior to being banned, Primatene Mist was the only asthma inhaler sold over the counter, and was indicated for the temporary relief of occasional mild asthma symptoms. Primatene mist also had the benefit of being affordable, at $20.00 per inhaler.

Prescription epinephrine in an injectable pen form has been in the news lately. Retailing as high as $467 per pen on average, the injectable form of epinephrine works the same way as the inhaler, relaxing the airway so that people in anaphylactic shock can breathe. In the hospital, we give 0.3cc of 1:1000 concentration of epinephrine for acute breathing problems. This amount is 1/3 of an amp that contains 3 doses, and costs about $11.00, representing quite a mark-up for those required to buy an epi-pen. It seems one could ask your physician for a prescription for the multi-dose ampule, and make your own epipen; a solution that might save lives.

A native plant useful for asthma sufferers is ephedra. Not to be confused with ephedrine alkaloids and pseudoephedrine that are currently semi-illegal and require a prescription, or at the very least subject to tracking and dosage limitations. Ephedra sinica is easy to grow, and has the benefit of expanding bronchial tubes, making breathing easier. Native Americans and Mormon pioneers relied on tea prepared from the ephedra plant, and it has the nickname Mormon tea. The Chinese call the plant ma huang. Ephedra eases symptoms of asthma by relaxing the trachea.

Growing ephedra is easy, and can it can easily be grown in a pot on your kitchen window ledge. When growing, it looks like grass, and for allergies, you can just clip off half an inch or so to ease breathing or quell allergy symptoms. When started from seed, you will have a small plant in about 5-6 weeks.

Ephedra in high doses does have side effects, such as fast heart beat, and a rise in blood pressure, but the small dose obtained from the natural plant (in small amounts) should not present any problems.

Note: Pseudoephedrine, found in drugs such as Sudafed, is one of the only drugs that effectively treats inner and middle ear congestion. Essentially a prescription medication, it can still be purchased over the counter, but requires photo identification for purchase.

Asthma quick help: Caffeine is chemically related to the drug theophylline that was used extensively in the past to treat asthma. In a review of several studies that have explored the effects of caffeine in asthma, the reviewers concluded that caffeine appears to improve airway function modestly in people with asthma for up to four hours. A quick home treatment for mild asthma is two cups of strong black coffee.

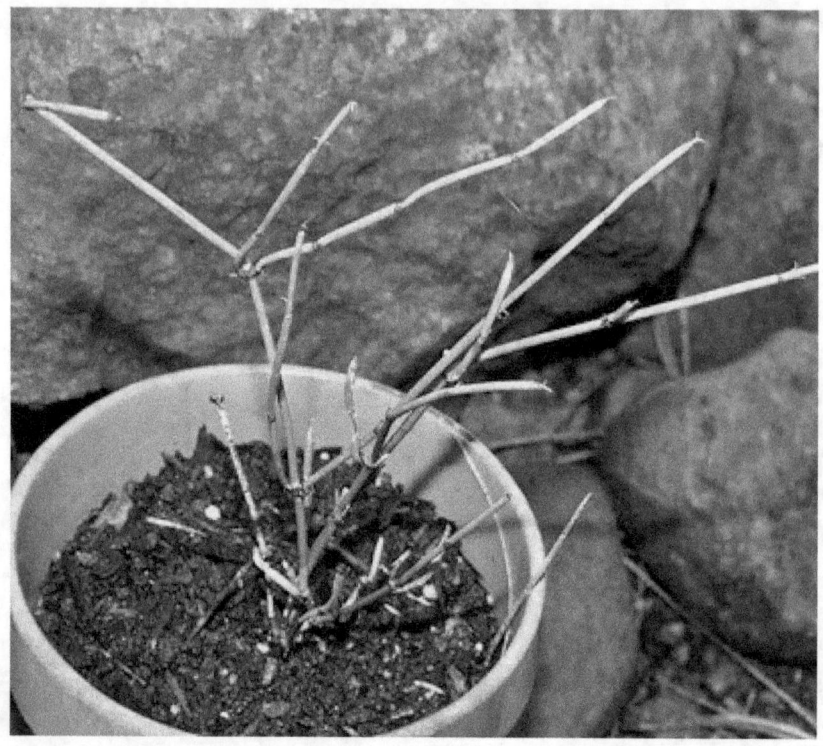

Ephedra grows like grass, and is happy growing in a small pot on a windowsill.

21 KAVA KAVA

Kava-Kava (Piper methysticum) is a plant known for its effect on anxiety, stress and restlessness. The medicinal part of the plant comes from the rhizome. In the South Pacific where the plant is native, including Hawaii, the root is often ingested by chewing, as saliva has been shown to strengthen the effect of chemicals contained in the plant. In Europe, Kava-Kava, commonly called Kava, is also consumed as a tea. In the United States, kava is very popular as a natural alternative to anti-anxiety drugs or sleeping pills. It is usually purchased as a powder, either in bulk or in capsules.

Anxiety

Dozens of studies have validated the effect on anxiety provided by Kava. In one study comparing the herb to Valium, it was shown to have similar effects. A recent study found the water-soluble extract of the kava plant to be safe and highly effective for the short-term treatment of anxiety, and hundreds of reviews on Amazon testify to its effectiveness. Kava has actual muscle relaxing effects, and has been shown to cause muscle relaxation to the point that animals that receive it fall out of revolving cages. It obviously shouldn't be taken prior to driving or operating equipment!

Epilepsy

The effect of kava on seizures is currently under investigation. Kava extract has been shown to have a protecting effect against convulsions. In clinical phase II trials, kava was effective in major clonic-tonic seizures, but when information about complications associated with high doses or long term use was presented, the clinical trials were discontinued. Kava protects against seizures by blocking sodium channels, thereby decreasing the conduction of seizure activity in certain areas of the brain, similar to Dilantin and other seizure drugs.

Other documented uses include treatment of asthma, for arthritis pain, and as a diuretic. When chewed, it numbs the lips and mouth, and food eaten after taking kava can't be tasted.

Toxicity

Kava abuse can have serious consequences. Overuse can cause weight loss, a distinctive scaly rash, and affect blood chemistry. Long-term use of Kava, even at recommended doses, has been show to result in liver toxicity. In 2003, there was a report of a previously healthy 14-year-old girl who was admitted to the hospital in liver failure. Treatment was unsuccessful, and she required a liver transplant after it was found her native liver showed cell death consistent with chemical hepatitis. When a thorough history was taken, she reported that during late August to mid-December 2000, she took two kava-containing products. Following the package directions, the girl took two capsules once daily of one product intermittently for about 44 days, and the second product two capsules once daily for 7 consecutive days at the beginning of the 4-month period. By December, she suffered from nausea, vomiting, decreased appetite, weight loss, and fatigue.

Not everyone agrees that Kava is toxic. When talking about the lifting of the German ban against Kava, a paper published in 2015 made the point that Kava has been used safely for more than 1000 years in social gatherings for the preparation of beverages with relaxing effects. Writer K. Kuchta went on to state, "During the colonial period, extract preparations found their way into Western medicinal systems, with experience especially concerning the treatment of situational anxiety dating back more than 100 years. It therefore came as a surprise when the safety of kava was suddenly questioned based on the observation of a series of case reports of liver toxicity in 1999 and 2000. These case reports ultimately led to a ban of kava products in Europe - a ban that has been contested because of the poor evidence of risks related to kava. Only recently, two German administrative courts decided that the decision of the regulatory authority to ban kava as a measure to ensure consumer safety was inappropriate and even associated with an increased risk due to the higher risk inherent to the therapeutic alternatives."

Everyone does agree that Kava is helpful for anxiety. Use your judgment if you try this herbal treatment for anxiety and/or sleeplessness, and avoid high doses or long-term use.

22 READ THE LABELS

By: Tamara Glascock

Trying to eat healthy can be a real challenge these days. Just because a label says 'organic' doesn't mean that all the ingredients are organic. Just because the label says 'made with natural ingredients' doesn't mean the whole product is made with natural ingredients.

You may have heard the adage, "if you can't pronounce it, you shouldn't be eating it," but that isn't necessarily true, either. For instance, cocos nucifera may not be easily recognized or pronounced, but it is simply coconut oil. Nothing nefarious there, right?

The safest option is to eat whole foods like fresh fruits and veggies, nuts and whole grains from GMO-free plants, and use only personal care products that contain ingredients you can easily recognize – or make your own! When that isn't really an option, familiarize yourself with some of the most dangerous ingredients and avoid them when possible.

How do we even begin to know what to look for when trying to eat healthy and avoid dangerous and unnatural products in our food and skin care products, short of earning a degree in science and learning Latin? While there is no easy answer, and it is almost impossible to list all of the ingredients to avoid, there are some general guidelines we can use when reading labels and choosing the safest products available.

When buying food products, avoid anything with artificial sweeteners like sorbitol, aspartame and sucralose. This also includes naturally-derived sweeteners like stevia, a sugar substitute that is often cut with things like carageenan, a product derived from a natural source (red algae), but causes severe negative reactions in the human body. Other food additives that are often found in processed foods and should be avoided include soybean oil, food dyes (especially Red 40, Yellow 5, and

Yellow 6), and MSG. MSG is often listed under several different names, including autolyzed yeast, calcium caseinate, yeast nutrient or extract, textured protein, gelatin, or hydrolyzed protein.

Unfortunately, dangerous ingredients aren't just contaminating our food. Personal hygiene products are laced with ingredients that are known to cause a whole host of health problems like eczema and skin problems, liver damage, cancer, brain and nervous system disorders, and much more. What many people do not realize is that our skin, the largest organ of the body, is capable of both releasing and absorbing toxins. That means that everything we place on our skin is being delivered into our bloodstream and carried throughout the rest of the body.

As with food labels, personal care labels leave a lot of room for misleading claims. When that shampoo says 'made with real fruit extract,' that simply means that it has a very small amount of 'real fruit extract.' It does not mean that is the main ingredient, or that the product does not contain many other ingredients that are dangerous to our health. To further complicate things, personal care products are not required to list every ingredient. There is a long list of ingredients that are considered 'incidental' by the FDA that aren't required to be listed on the label.

In the case of personal care products, paying attention to what *isn't* in the product can be just as important as what *is* in the product. Look for products that are fragrance-free. Avoid products that claim to be anti-bacterial. Avoid anything containing polyethylene glycol (PEG). A few other ingredients to avoid include; 1,4-dioxane (any ingredient that contains 'eth' are most likely a version of 1,4-dioxane), parabens, phthalates, methylisothiazolinone (MIT), triclosan, and propylene glycol.

Take time to read the labels! It is surely worth your time.

23 IODINE

Recently I had the pleasure of working with a physician who practiced holistic medicine. For many of his patients, potassium iodide was prescribed.

It is estimated that more than 11 percent of all American have moderate to severe iodine deficiency. Another 36 percent are considered mildly iodine deficient. Iodine levels have significantly dropped in the United States in recent decades due to several factors, including bromine exposure, the lack of iodine-rich foods, and fluoridated drinking water.

The Japanese ingest almost 90 times more iodine than Americans, largely due to their consumption of seafood. The Japanese also have the lowest rates of cancer in the world. While the typical Japanese citizen consumes 13800 mcg. of iodine, in the United States, the Recommended Daily Allowance (RDA) for iodine is 150 micrograms daily for everybody over the age of 14. The RDA for children ages 1-8 is 90/mcg every day, and for ages 9-13 is 120/mcg every day. If you're pregnant or breastfeeding, it is recommended that you get 290/mcg every day.

Sources of iodine

One source of iodine comes from salt to which iodine has been added, i.e. iodized salt. Not all salt is equal, so it is essential to check your labels. In order to get enough iodine from salt, you would be putting your blood pressure at risk. Fortunately, iodine is also found in saltwater fish, shellfish, eggs, fish, cranberries, navy beans, organic cheese and potatoes, yogurt, soy sauce, and sea vegetables such as kelp or seaweed.

Role of Iodine in the body

Iodine is essential for proper functioning of the thyroid, and maintains its ability to make important thyroid hormones. Eating foods rich in iodine ensures the thyroid is able to manage metabolism, detoxification, growth and development. Lack of iodine may lead to enlargement of the thyroid gland, with symptoms like lethargy, fatigue, weakness of the immune system, a slow metabolism and associated weight gain, and goiters.

Importance of Iodine in pregnancy

Physiological changes in pregnancy result in increased iodine demand, which may not be met in areas of mild-to-moderate iodine deficiency or borderline sufficiency. When a woman is pregnant, she is the only source of thyroid hormones for her unborn child, and insufficient iodine intake can have adverse effects on the development of the fetus. Iodine deficiency is a major cause of brain damage if not corrected early in pregnancy. Research published February 2017 in the Journal of Nutrition concluded that "Iodine deficiency early in the life cycle-the 'first 1000 days'-can cause hypothyroidism and irreversibly impair neuromotor development."

Iodine allergy

People who have undergone diagnostic tests may have an allergic reaction to the dye, causing them to be labeled with an iodine allergy. Most contrast media contains iodine, as it shows up well on x-ray. There are several studies showing that the allergy may not be due to iodine, but rather to a component in the dye. Many experts feel the term "iodine allergy" should be changed to contrast media allergy, because it is potentially dangerous and can decrease the quality of radiology exams.

Iodine and Radiation

In the wake of the nuclear fallout at Fukushima, Japan, there was a shortage of potassium iodide as people attempted to protect themselves from radiation, including radioactive iodine. With enough natural iodine in the body, radioactive iodine has nowhere to bind, and will be excreted. As the thyroid is particularly affected by radioactive iodine, those not protected are very predisposed to develop thyroid cancer. In fact, the rates of thyroid cancers in both humans and animals are on the increase on the west coast.

24 WATCH WHAT YOU COOK WITH

Food absorbs elements of any container in which it is cooked or stored. This can have positive or detrimental effects on our health, and should be considered in any healthy lifestyle.

Teflon

Introduced in the 1960's, Teflon was all the rage. Everyone wanted the nonstick pots and pans. The problem is, that when heated to high temperatures, this coating creates hazardous fumes that cause cancer and birth defects in animals. DuPont, the inventor of Teflon, has denied charges brought by the federal government regarding the hazardous effects of Teflon. DuPont also maintains that it has no legal obligations to report their research findings to the federal government, claiming that components of Teflon posed no danger to humans at past or current levels and therefore, the information did not have to be reported to the EPA.

In regards to Teflon, owners of pet birds can attest to the canary in the coalmine scenario. In a single year in Chicago, a veterinarian recorded 296 bird deaths in 105 cases involving Teflon cookware. A review of the literature shows that Teflon can indeed be lethal at normal cooking temperatures.   Bird deaths generally occur within minutes after exposure to the fumes, due to what has been termed Teflon toxicosis. DuPont claims that its coating remains intact indefinitely at 500°F, but independent reports find that nonstick coatings are a risk if they are heated to temperatures greater than 350°C, as can easily happen if an empty pan is left on a burner. In this case, the coatings can give off irritating or poisonous fumes.

Aluminum

Aluminum is lightweight, inexpensive, and a good conductor of heat, but many folks are getting rid of their aluminum cookware. Ingesting aluminum provides no benefit to the body, but has been associated with Alzheimer's Disease due to unusually high levels of aluminum found in the brains of Alzheimer patients at autopsy. Cooking with aluminum is estimated to add 2 mg of the soft metal to your diet daily. The World Health Organization estimates that adults can consume more than 50 milligrams of aluminum daily without harm, but people with severe kidney disease can retain higher amounts of aluminum in their bodies, leading to dementia, anemia or bone disease. During cooking, aluminum is absorbed most easily from old and worn pots and pans. Aluminum is a poor choice for food storage, because the longer food is cooked or stored in aluminum, the greater the amount absorbed. Acidic foods, such as tomato containing products and leafy vegetables, absorb the most aluminum. Because aluminum is known to cause lung damage if large amounts are inhaled, and is also considered a neurotoxin, poisonous to the brain and nervous system, the safety of dietary aluminum and this cookware remains controversial.

Safer Choices

We are careful about the foods we choose, reading labels, purchasing fresh produce, avoiding GMO's, and choosing organic as much as possible, but all these healthy choices are defeated if food is not prepared and stored properly. Using well-seasoned cast-iron, stainless steel, or glass cookware is not only safe, but can actually enhance the nutritional quality of food.

Iron Cookware

Iron cookware has been shown to greatly improve the nutritional status of vegetarians who often don't ingest enough iron. A study published in the July 1986 issue of the *Journal of the American Dietetic Association* found that cooking in cast iron skillets added significant amounts of iron to 20 foods tested. Researchers found that the iron content of three ounces of applesauce increased from 0.35 mg to 7.3 mg and scrambled eggs increased from 1.49 mg to 4.76 mg of iron.

Iron cookware may not work well when cooking tomatoes as the acidic nature of the tomatoes can discolor the end protect, and give a slightly metallic taste. It's okay for cooking briefly, but not for simmering on the stove for hours. Iron cookware is also not recommended for deep-frying as iron can accelerate the oxidation of fat and cause it to become rancid.

Stainless Steel

When cooking tomatoes, stainless steel is a good choice. Stainless steel is chemically inert, so not very much is absorbed into your food. Steel is more expensive, and doesn't conduct heat as well as aluminum, thus "copper clad" stainless steel cookware was developed. In order to determine if a pan is steel or aluminium, remember that steel is a heavier metal, and aluminum scratches and pits easier. Also, steel is often magnetic (not always), but aluminum never is.

25 BROMELAIN AND PINEAPPLE

This darn cough

Have a hacking cough that just won't go away? Don't want to give your child cough syrup with possibly harmful ingredients? There is a natural solution – pineapple! Adding honey to pineapple makes for an even more powerful cough suppressant, even healing conditions like thick phlegm and irritation of the throat that can lead to chronic cough.

Usually cough is due to a viral illness, and is self-limiting. A chronic, irritating cough can result from several causes. It can become so intense that it leads both the patient and their family to exhaustion. Often, chronic cough is due to thickened saliva that comes with conditions like allergies, chronic sinus drainage, colds and flu, inhaling irritants in the atmosphere, bronchitis, COPD, Parkinson's Disease, emphysema and heart failure, to name a few. With most of these, it is inflammation or the presence of excess or thick saliva that makes a cough chronic and irritating.

Over the counter cough syrup can bring risks, especially to childen. Dextromethorphan (DMX) and Benedryl are often used in cough preparations, but can be dangerous, and natural remedies often work better for children. DMX has been used by teens to "get high," and deaths have been reported. What most parents don't realize when administering cough medication containing DMX is that fact that approximately 10% of children do not possess the proper enzymes needed to effectively metabolize the drug, so even when taken at recommended dosages, it can still be fatal. Benadryl isn't very safe in children either, and can cause effects on the central nervous system like sedation or stimulation, leading to seizures. A clinical study in children found that half a teaspoon of honey given before sleep showed better result in cough relief than either Benadryl or DMX.

Bromelain

Bromelain, a mixture of enzymes capable of breaking down proteins, is found in all parts of the pineapple plant. Bromelain is capable of dissolving thick mucus, the usual cause of a chronic, irritating cough. In addition to dissolving mucus, bromelain also has anti-inflammatory effects on the respiratory tract.

The World Health Organization has listed honey as a safe treatment for cough in upper respiratory tract infections in children. Honey has been shown to have antioxidant, antibacterial, antifungal, antiviral, anti-inflammatory and anti-tumor actions. In one study, researchers concluded, "The combination of pineapple extract with honey may present a breakthrough in the symptomatic treatment, possibly by blocking triggering mechanisms of cough due to viral or irritative conditions."

Other effects

While the anti-inflammatory effect of pineapple helps to decrease the production of mucus in the airway, in healthy humans eating pineapple has been shown to help several autoimmune and inflammatory diseases, including ulcerative colitis, multiple sclerosis and respiratory tract infections. In Europe, bromelain is used to treat sinus and nasal swelling following ear, nose, and throat surgery or trauma. Bromelain may also relieve the swelling and inflammation caused by hay fever.

Side effects

The bromelain content of raw pineapple is responsible for the sore mouth feeling often experienced when eating it, as the same enzymes that break down mucus can break down the sensitive tissues in the mouth. Otherwise, pineapple is very safe, with only a mild and self-limiting allergic reaction in a patient allergic to pineapple.

26 CLEAVERS

Galium aparine, known by the common name "Cleavers" is a native plant, not only in Missouri, but in much of the world. It gets its name from the hooked bristles on its stems, seeds and leaves that make it cling to objects it comes in contact with, including other plants. The ability to cling on to adjacent plants enables it to climb through dense undergrowth into full sunlight. It grows just about everywhere.

Cleavers belong to the Rubiaceae, or madder family; also the family of coffee, quinine, and gardenia, with many of the same benefits. The plant has narrow, lance-shaped leaves that are rough to the touch with backward pointing prickles. The stem is square (although not in the mint family like most square-stemmed plants), and it can grow up to 6 or more feet in length. It blooms from April through September, producing tiny white flowers.

Nutritional value

Cleavers are edible, but not very tasty when eaten raw. The bristles can stick in your mouth and throat, a problem solved with cooking, which is why they are mostly used as a potherb or added to soups. Eating the plant as a vegetable has been reported to aid in weight loss. The plant provides beneficial Vitamin C. Seed from the Cleavers plant is considered an excellent substitute for coffee. When dried and roasted, seeds from the Cleavers plant have the same flavor, but less caffeine than regular coffee. The plant also provides food for the larvae of several butterfly species.

Medicinal Uses

The Cleavers plant has been used in natural medicine for centuries. It can be used both internally and externally to treat skin problems, and for a general detoxification of the body. The plant also acts as a diuretic. The active ingredients of the plant include organic acids, flavonoids, tannins, fatty acids, glycoside asperuloside, gallotannic acid and citric acid. The plant is of great interest to the pharmaceutical industry, and sells for $25.00 a pound on Amazon with dozens of five-star reviews for its effects.

Detox agent

The plant is able to absorb toxic chemicals, and its diuretic action helps to flush them out of the body via the urinary tract. In fact, the Cleaver plant is so efficient at this; it can be planted on contaminated farmland to take toxic chemicals out of the soil. Studies on farmland contaminated with Cadmium show that Cleavers are considered a hyper-accumulator, drawing cadmium out of the soil very efficiently. Cadmium exerts toxic effects on the kidney, the skeletal system and the respiratory system and is classified as a human carcinogen. (Cadmium can occur naturally, but more often from mining, smelting and refining of non-ferrous metals.)

Skin problems

The Cleavers plant is also used to treat skin problems such as oily skin, eczema and psoriasis. A poultice made from the Cleavers herb can be used for wounds, skin ulcers, and as a drawing agent. It acts as an astringent to tighten the skin. Drinking tea made from the plant is reported to clear up acne. When used as a hair rinse, it is said to promote hair growth.

Urinary System

The plant can be used to treat bladder and urinary problems. It acts as an astringent in the bladder, and helps to reduce calcium deposits. It has been used to decrease frequency and severity of gallbladder attacks.

To make a medicinal tea, add 3 heaping tablespoons of dried herb to 1 pint of boiling water, and let steep 10 minutes. Drink as desired.

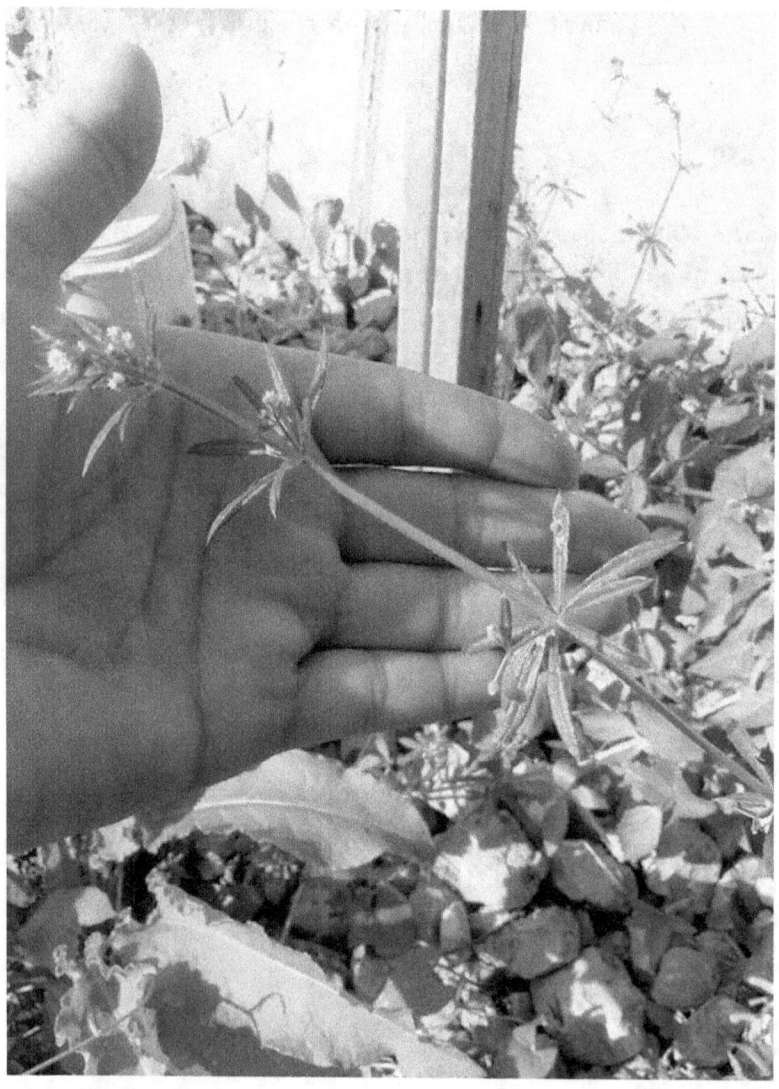

Cleavers are easy to identify. They have a square stem and "cleave" to your hand when you touch them.

27 WHITE CLOVER

While red clover has been extensively researched and its nutritional and women's health properties are well known, other forms of clover are just now getting attention from pharmaceutical companies. For example, sweet clover possesses significant amounts of coumarin, which is bio-identical to the blood thinner warfarin.

White clover, Latin name *Trifolium repens, has nutritional and medicinal uses all its own. White clover was originally native to Europe, West Asia and Northern Africa. It is sometimes called Dutch clover, because it was first cultivated in Holland, but white clover now grows all around the world. The flowers are loaded with nectar,* making it an excellent bee plant. White clover honey is white or nearly white; very mild flavored and doesn't tend to granulate.

When planted in a field, White clover has nitrogen-fixing abilities, acting to improve the soil. It can thrive in many different type of soils, at different pH levels. When white clover grows in an apple orchard, it has been found to improve the flavor of the fruit and extend the storage period.

Nutritional purposes

When used for food, all parts of the plant, including leaves, flowers, seedpods and roots are edible. The leaves are most tender and tasty when picked before the clover blooms, and can be used raw in a salad, or cooked like spinach.

White clover is 25% crude protein by weight, and includes significant amounts of calcium, phosphorus, magnesium, sodium and potassium.

Dried white clover leaves can be used as a vanilla substitute, and flower heads can be dried and powderized, then added to flour to both extend it and to add nutrients.

Medicinal Uses

For medicinal purposes, the leaves and flowers are used. Native Americans used the leaves in an herbal tea to treat cough, colds and fevers. In Europe, the tea was consumed to treat gout and rheumatism. Clover works well as a diuretic, reducing inflammation in cases of gout. White clover is also considered to reduce inflammation due to arthritis. The isoflavones found in red clover have been found beneficial in reducing bone loss and menopausal symptoms in healthy women. White clover does not have the same properties or health benefits as red clover, but still has limited medicinal use.

White clover contains the chemicals biochanin A, urolic acid, betulinic acid and beta-sitosterol, chemicals found to work as antihelmintics, also known as wormers. Because it is effective against tapeworms, medications are being developed from the plant to treat worms in farm animals. Obviously white clover is a good pasture plant when raising horses, sheep or goats.

Anti-oxidant

Like many clovers, white clover contains estrogen-like compounds, which have cancer-preventative and antioxidant activity.

Neuroprotection

In a study involving the Pikuni-Blackfete tribe in western Montana, studies were carried out on white clover to evaluate its effect on Parkinson's disease related symptoms. The goal was to identify medicinal plants that would be affordable for the Native American community. In the study, tribal healers and local people were interviewed on the Blackfeet Indian reservation. Plant samples were collected, and water extracts were produced for subsequent analysis. A sample of botanical extracts was tested for the ability to prevent or slow nerve degeneration in Parkinson's disease. White clover was found to protect the nervous system from toxic agents, while garlic and serviceberry prevented actual cell death.

Even though red clover has already established a great reputation for both its nutritional and pharmaceutical properties, look for the discovery of more uses for white clover.

28 MAKE YOUR OWN CLEANING PRODUCTS

Did you know that Pine Sol no longer contains pine? If you look at the ingredients, you will find ingredients like alcohol ethoxylates, glycolic acid, dimethicone, distearates, sodium C14-17 secondary alkyl sulfonate, and other chemical equations.

It is easy to make great cleaning products with natural ingredients you may be throwing in the trash. The first rule of making your own products is to save your empty spray bottles and other containers to use for storage and dispensing the product. (*Note: Never mix ammonia in a bleach container or vice versa. Combining these products produces a toxic gas, something this writer found out the hard way as a teenager.)

To make your own Pine-sol (effective against many types of bacteria and viruses, including influenza A), collect and wash a handful of fresh green pine needles. Crush them to start to release the oils, then soak in enough rubbing alcohol to cover. Let stand for a week, and then strain off the solution. Add 1 part of pine extract to 5 parts of water. Store in a well washed used spray bottle, and you are ready to clean and disinfect with no worry of harm to your pets or yourself.

Counter Cleaners

The power of citrus is pretty well known, and is a common additive to many cleaning products. The easiest way to make citrus cleaner is by putting your lemon or orange peels in a clean container with about a quart of water. Let it sit for about two weeks, and you will have an excellent cleaner and degreaser, ideal for cleaning the top of the stove.

To make turbo citrus cleaner, replace the water in the above recipe with vinegar. This is a super cleaner for really tough jobs. You can spray it on a messy surface, let it sit a few minutes, and then easily wipe off with a cloth.

Garbage Disposal Deodorizer

If you don't use all of your citrus peels to make counter cleaner, save a few to run through your garbage disposal. Dry or fresh, citrus peels will degrease your garbage disposal, and leave it with a pleasant, citrusy scent.

Window Cleaner

Forget Windex, a weak ammonia solution will make your windows sparkling clean. Use old newspapers instead of paper towels for a sparkling clean, lint-free shine. While you're at it, ammonia is the best thing to shine up stainless steel sinks, coffee pots, refrigerators and other appliances. While there are methods of making homemade ammonia, they are fairly complicated. Since ammonia is so inexpensive, it is worthwhile picking up a quart of it. Some folks prefer to use vinegar for cleaning windows.

Limescale Dissolver

If you have well water, you likely have limescale deposits on your sink and toilet fixtures. Vinegar effortlessly dissolves the deposits in minutes, and nothing else works better. To make your own vinegar, take clean apple peels and put them in a glass container. Completely cover with water, cover with a cloth and place in a cool damp place for 3 weeks, Voila! Vinegar. There may be some mold on the top, just scoop it off and discard, the liquid vinegar will be fine, even for cooking use.

Mold Eraser

You can't completely eradicate mold with bleach, but a simple recipe will erase 99.9% of mold, including black mold, and is non-toxic to people and pets. Add TSP (tri-sodium phosphate, available at most hardware stores) to get rid of the mold/mildew and keep it from coming back. A good, strong, all-around solution is four quarts of fresh water, one quart of bleach, 2/3 cup of TSP, and 1/3 cup of powdered laundry detergent. Do not use liquid detergents in combination with bleach. Just wipe down surfaces with a cloth, and all mold will come off. You can also put it in an old Windex bottle and spray it on hard to reach places, like moldy closet corners.

Laundry Soap

The following is my grandmother's recipe for laundry soap, found on a handwritten note in her 1930's cookbook.

For washing and bleaching, put 4 lb. of washing soda in a vessel with one gallon of weather. Put on the fire and boil 10 minutes. Then add 1 lb. of chloride of lime. Then cold strain and keep in a jug lightly corked. Put a handful of soap chips in hot water. Then add 1/2 cup of the bleacher. Either soak clothes over Sunday, or wash in half an hour after soaking, but do not boil clothes.

Making your own cleaning products will not only save money, but is healthier for your home.

29 OX-EYE DAISY

Leucanthemum vulgare, also known as ox-eye daisy, is blooming everywhere in the Ozarks right now. A perennial herb, the ox-eye daisy is native to Europe, but grows throughout the world. The blooms are the brightest and freshest in mid-May, but are still vibrant until the end of June. The flower heads have a protective base, a ring of green brackets that also serve to protect the flower from insects biting into the nectar it contains.

Nutrition

In Italy, the leaves are added to salads, but the plant is not very palatable as it produces an acrid juice. This juice protects the plant, acting as an insecticide. Eating it won't hurt you, but it's not very tasty.

Medicinal Use

In traditional medicine, a tea made from extract of the whole plant is used to treat asthma and bronchitis. Crushing the leaves and stem releases an antifungal and antibacterial agent that can be applied to skin lesions. Herbalists also value the plant for its antispasmodic, diuretic and tonic properties. A fluid extract of the root can be used to treat night sweats; add 15 to 60 drops to a glass of water. The active ingredients include alkaloids, flavonoids and phenolic chemicals. The volatile oil showed free-radical-scavenging and antifungal effects. As discussed before, free radicals are unpaired molecules in the body that are unstable, and harm healthy cells. They are also a major source of aging. Anti-oxidants neutralize these free radicals, protecting the body from their toxic effects.

Jaundice

There are many reports in historical literature about the use of ox-tail daisy in treating jaundice. Jaundice, of course, occurs to dysfunction of the liver, gallbladder or pancreas. The leaves and stems can be boiled, then sweetened with honey and enjoyed like a tea.

External Use

Applied to the skin, ox-tail daisy works heal wounds, bruises and other skin conditions. Extract from the plant can be made into a lotion or salve, or the leaves can be bruised and applied directly to swollen tissue and used to ease the pain of sciatica or gout.

Soil Remediation

Sites with crude oil pollution have been successfully treated by planting ox-eye daisies. The roots of the plant become colonized by a type of fungus that doesn't hurt the plant, but loves to eat hydrocarbons. The lowest hydrocarbon reading in contaminated soil has been recorded six months after the ox-eye daisy was planted. Think of the difference between a contaminated piece of land, and one covered with beautiful daisies.

Whatever the application, Ox-Eye Daisies are safe, with the exceptional case of contact dermatitis reported from contact with the plant.

Companion Plants

When you're out exploring native plants, you may also find a very cool surprise growing in the area of the ox-tail daisy – Cat's Claw, also known as Sensitive Briar. Touch the leaves, and they put on a little show for you as rows of them close up tightly.

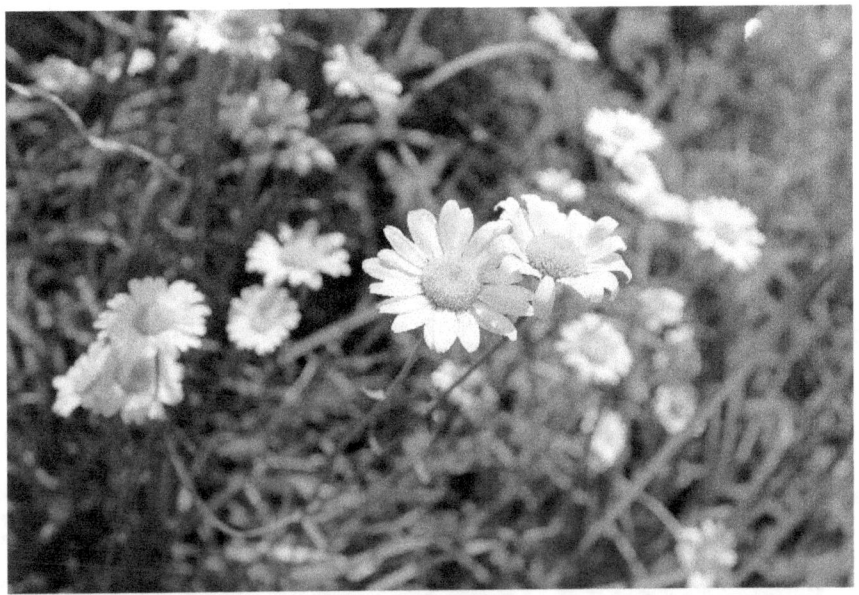

Beautiful Ox Eye Daisies are dotting the landscape in the Ozarks.

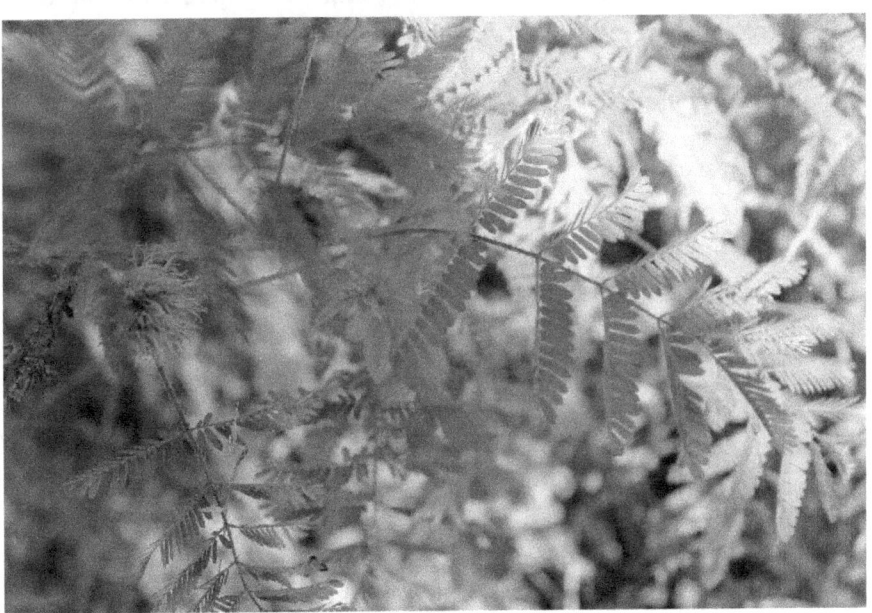

Sensitive Brier has sensitive leaves that react to your soft touch.

30 BORON ISN'T BORING

A reader stopped into the Licking News last week, interested in learning more about boron. As it turns out, the trace mineral boron is an absolutely essential micronutrient, essential for plant, animal and human health.

Boron primary role involves bone development and regeneration. It also promotes healing of wounds, production and metabolism of Vitamin D, calcium and magnesium. In addition to all this, boron can alleviate arthritis, improve brain function, and prevent cancer.

Boron is banned as a food additive in the United States and Thailand. The absence of studies showing harm, compared with research showing the beneficial effects, support taking a boron supplement of 3 mg/day.

Bone growth and repair

Boron is essential for healthy bones and helps to develop new bone tissue. It also prevents calcium loss and bone demineralization. Research has proven that boron supplements improve bone strength in both the inner and outer parts of the bone. Boron also helps to repair bones by speeding up the development of osteoblasts, specialized immature bone cells that join together to make new bone and knit broken bones together. Boron does this in part by helping the body to use calcium more efficiently.

Wound Healing

Boron doesn't just help bones heal; it also significantly improves wound healing. In one study, applying 3% boric acid solution to deep wounds helped them heal about 60% faster. Another study found the healing effects of boron were due to direct actions on enzymes involved in wound healing, and like with bone, aid the development of fibroblasts, cells that provide the framework for wound healing.

Regulation of Sex Hormones

A study from 2011 found that after only one week on daily boron supplements of 6 mg/day, healthy males found a significant increase in free testosterone. In women, Boron can reduce the severity and duration of menstrual pain through anti-inflammatory effects. In postmenopausal women, boron increased estradiol and testosterone levels. Estradiol is important for women's bone health.

Prevention of Vitamin D Deficiency

When boron is given to people with vitamin D deficiency, (worse during the winter months due to less sunlight exposure), Vitamin D levels rise significantly, an average of 20%. Also, some people just don't seem to be able to retain Vitamin D. When boron supplements are added, even Vitamin D "nonresponders" see their levels rise.

Magnesium absorption

Many people are deficient in magnesium, partially due to phosphate fertilizers that leach magnesium from the body. 60% of magnesium in the human body is found in the bones, and magnesium is necessary for the formation of new bone cells. Boron improves both the absorption of magnesium into the body, and helps it deposit into the bones.

Anti-inflammatory

Multiple studies have proven the effectiveness of boron in the treatment of osteoarthritis. Looking at people around the world, in areas where boron intake is less than 1 mg/dl, the rate of arthritis ranges from 20% - 70%. However, in areas of the world where the average boron intake is 3 – 10 mg/dl, the incidence of arthritis is less than 10%, or even non-existent.

Brain activity

Not enough boron in the diet has been linked to decreased electrical activity in the brain. Research studies have shown that humans suffering from boron deprivation tested poorly on tasks of motor speed and dexterity, attention, and short-term memory. Boron helps the body to detox from fluoride poisoning, a serious issue that results in weakened bones and lowered IQ in children.

Anti-cancer effects

Several studies have shown that boron has anti-cancer properties. In a national study, the risk of prostate cancer was 52% lower in men who consumed at least 1.8 mg/dl of boron per day. Boron, in the form of boric acid, has been show to decrease the size of prostate tumors in animal studies. Other cancers benefitted from boron include cervical and lung cancers. Boron based drugs are being developed to treat multiple myeloma and non-Hodgkin's lymphoma. Forget the controversial drug Gardasil – boron interferes in the life cycle of human papilloma virus, thought to be the main cause of cervical cancer. Turkey has soil very rich in boron and an extremely low incidence of cervical cancer.

Foods High in Boron

Avocado is the top food in the boron department, followed by peanut butter, dry peanuts and prune juice. When taking a supplement, 3 mg daily is the recommended dose.

31 MAKING POULTICES

By: Tamara Glascock

Herbal poultices are one of the oldest forms of herbal medicine for good reason. They are simple, highly effective, and are used to treat a wide variety of issues. Poultices have been used to treat bruises, wounds, broken bones, skin diseases, constipation, organ congestion, and even many chronic conditions that don't respond well to conventional medical treatments. They are as easy to assemble in an emergency, and the results are most often immediate.

To prepare a simple poultice that works well to combat against bites and stings, or on wounds to help staunch bleeding and draw tissues together, find a nice plantain leaf and lightly chew it until it is moist. Human saliva activates the medicinal components of herbs, making this especially useful in field medicine. Place the chewed plantain leaf directly over the bite/sting. You will find instant relief from pain and itching.

When you are using a poultice that will need to cover a larger area, or will need to be left on for a longer period of time, the process is much the same, but requires a few more ingredients. You will need the following:

Plant material – fresh plant material is best, but dried will work. You want your plant material as small as possible to make it easier to work with. Fresh herbs can be cut into small bits or crushed with a mortar and pestle. Dried herbs can be ground into a powder. Roots can be especially difficult to use in poultices. I have found that grinding them up makes them much more manageable.

You will need:

- Liquid – apple cider vinegar, a carrier oil such as olive or sesame oil, or distilled water are the best options.
- A piece of plastic large enough to cover the desired area. We have used plastic wrap, recycled grocery bags and plastic baggies. The plastic is used to help hold in the heat and keep it from dripping all over your clothes/bedding.
- A piece of natural fiber cloth slightly larger than the plastic. Cotton, wool or hemp are all great options.
- A hot pack, hot water bottle or heating pad. Any source of heat will work fine, but damp heat is preferable.

To prepare the poultice, add just enough of the liquid to moisten the plant material. It should be damp, but not dripping. Gently warm it until it is slightly above your normal body temp. Warmer is better, but be careful not to make it hot enough to burn you. You do not want to use the microwave for this. The best way is to place the mixture in a heat-safe glass vessel, then place the vessel in hot water until the desired temperature is reached.

Place the mixture over the affected area. For larger areas, extend the mixture out slightly past the edges of the area being treated. Cover the mixture with the plastic, then place the material over the plastic. Place the hot pack over the cloth. You do not want to let the poultice cool until you are ready to remove it.

Leave the poultice in place for at least 30 minutes, though an hour or more is best.

After you remove the poultice, wash the area mild soap and water, or a mixture of ¼ cup apple cider vinegar and 1 cup warm water.

32 DOCK

Dock is abundant everywhere, with over 200 varieties. A member of the buckwheat family and also related to rhubarb, many varieties of dock are not native to Missouri, but can be found here after being introduced to North America from Eurasia and North Africa. It has both food and medicinal values, and is a good plant to know.

Nutritional Value

There are many edible docks in the *Rumex* genus, some native and some introduced. Commonly found Curly dock and bitter dock are introduced species, while willow dock and western dock are natives. The flavor varies among the species, but Curly dock is the top pick for salads.

3.5 ounces of raw dock have just 22 calories, but 2 grams of protein. Dock also contains vitamins A, C, thiamine, riboflavin, niacin and folate in addition to important minerals calcium, iron, magnesium, manganese, phosphorus, potassium and zinc. While a nutritious choice for humans, dock isn't so great for livestock. Curly dock in particular is toxic to goats, cattle and sheep. During the Great Depression, a variety of dock plants helped to keep folks from starving. Dock is often considered a nuisance weed, but several varieties are grown for their tender, edible leaves. The leaves also have other uses; such as broad leaf dock, also known as butter dock, which was used to wrap home-made butter and keep it fresh.

Medicinal Use

Curled (or Curly) dock is a popular member of the dock family with a long history as a domestic herb. All parts of the plant are useful, but the root is most active for medicinal use. An extract of the plant is used to treat a variety of chronic skin diseases, and the root can be mashed and prepared as a poultice or dried and used as a dusting powder on sores and lesions..

The root is most potent when harvested in early spring, but can be dried for later use. Although a preparation made from the leaves works as a gentle laxative, the seed is used to treat diarrhea. A homeopathic remedy used to treat a nagging tickling cough, also described as "incessant, violent coughing," is made from the fresh root, harvested in the autumn before frost has touched the plant. Western herbalists use the root to treat anemia, as it is high in iron.

Extracts from the leaves and seeds have antibacterial action against *staph aureus* and *B. subtilis*, properties that may explain its use as a treatment for many skin problems, In India, the roots and seeds are used to make toothpaste.

A tea made from the root is used to treat tapeworms and roundworms, likely effective because the contain oxymethyl anthraquinone compounds, also used to treat a variety of diseases due to parasites.

Another reason to love and respect the lowly dock plant is the fact it is also a food plant for members of the Lepidoptera species that includes the Monarch Butterfly and Luna Moth.

Cautions:

Dock can contain quite high levels of oxalic acid, accounting for the acidic lemon flavor in the leaves of many of the dock varieties. Fine in small quantities, the leaves should not be eaten raw in large amounts since the oxalic acid can potentially aggravate gout or cause kidney stones. The oxalic acid content will be reduced if the plant is cooked.

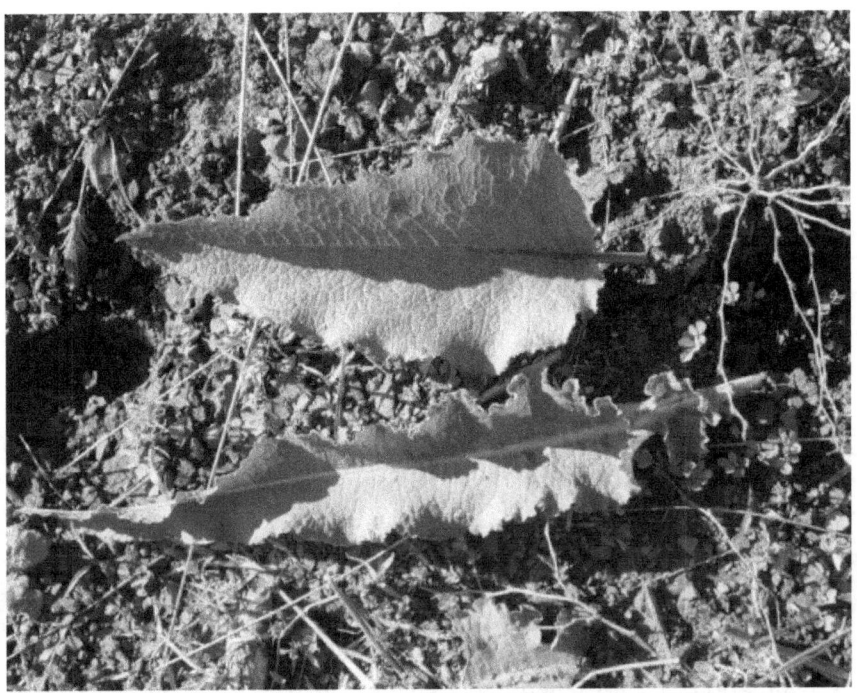

2 types of dock - upper is Broadleaf, also known as bitter dock; and lower is the popular Curly Dock – shaped like a lance with a curly edge.

33 FASTING THE EASY WAY

Many animals and humans alike alternate periods of eating with periods of fasting, Unless you wake up during the night to eat, most people effortlessly fast at least 6 – 8 hours nightly.

We all know that good things happen while we sleep. The fasting period is one of those good things because even one overnight fast results in lower concentrations of fats, insulin and glucose in the bloodstream - a more prefect state of health, and reason why lab specimens are ideally drawn after a period of fasting.

Research in animals highlights the importance of meshing fasting cycles with circadian rhythm. Consuming food during "normal eating times" protects against obesity, elevated insulin levels, fatty liver and inflammation. It's no wonder that night-shift workers have such high levels of obesity!

Other good things that happen with fasting are a state of ketosis that happens after a period of fasting when the body does not take in enough carbohydrates to replenish energy stores. The brain starts burning ketones to more directly use energy from the body's fat stores, and reserves glucose only for absolute needs. This avoids depleting our body's protein store in the muscles, and has many positive effects, including protecting the brain, slowing the effects of aging, and weight loss.

Despite what we may have heard all of our lives, skipping breakfast and prolonging our night-time fast (and state of ketosis) is related to a lower incidence of all diseases and longer life spans as compared with breakfast eaters.

Prolonged Fasting

Calorie restriction has been shown to have profound anti-aging benefits.

The problem is that total fasting and restricting calories are hard programs to stick with due to non-stop hunger. It is interesting that this persistent hunger is purely psychological. You can even prove this to yourself. Have you ever eaten a full, satisfying meal, not feeling the least amount of hunger, when a commercial comes on with people eating and suddenly feeling compelled to eat?

In one study conducted over 2 days, two sets of meals were given to subjects, one containing calories and one without. There was no difference in brain performance, activity, sleep or mood when the subjects and researchers were unaware of the calorie content of the meals. We have lots of clues, other than the body's need for food, that trigger our eating habits. Fortunately, there is another way to fast that provides all the health benefits of prolonged fasting, and anyone can reap the benefits.

Time Restricted Fasting

As previously mentioned, we all fast at night. When the period of fasting is lengthened to at least 16 hours, for example 6 pm to 10 am, no matter the total calorie intake, there are documented positive health effects. This form of fasting is simple and easy to follow, and since your meals are only a few hours away from your sleep time, hunger is not much of an issue. The long-term effect of time restricted fasting, which prolongs the period that that body is in ketosis, has been found to be strongly neuro-protective and beneficial for brain function, including those with Alzheimer's disease. Other health outcomes from fasting include significant weight loss, decreased fat, improved metabolic function, reduction in fasting glucose levels and lipid levels and lower incidence of cardiac disease and cancer.

Not just physical, benefits derived from fasting include improved mood self-confidence and decreased tension, anger and fatigue.

Give time restricted fasting a try for one week. You can expect greater mental clarity, and probably some weight loss.

34 BLACK CHOKEBERRY

(*Aronia melanocarpia*)

Black chokeberry, well known to folks in the Ozarks, is a native plant that originated in eastern parts of North America. Presently the plant is endangered in Missouri, so care should be taken with the plant if you are fortunate enough to have some on your property. It is a native plant, usually found in moist woodlands. The berries can be used to make jams, jellies, juice and wine. They are also used in nutritional supplements, and even used to color other foods. The berries have naturally high pectin content perfect for making jelly. And guess what? The plant has no thorns, a definite plus for berry pickers! Unlike choke cherry, the fruits of chokeberry aren't bitter; one way to distinguish the two.

Chokeberries have potent medicinal effects on intestinal issues, liver diseases, cancer and inflammation, to name a few. Like all berry crops, the fruit is also a great source of antioxidants.

Source of Nutrition

Chokeberries are full of bio-available vitamin A and C, potassium, calcium, and magnesium. Because of the abundance of important vitamins and minerals they contain, chokeberries are considered superior to many of the more common berries. The berries ripen as early as mid-July, but the best harvest dates are often the end of August or early September.

Antioxidants

Chokeberries are full of antioxidants. Antioxidants are important because they scavenge and destroy free radicals, compounds in the body that cause premature aging and can lead to chronic diseases like atherosclerosis, inflammation, cancer, and neurodegenerative disease. As an antioxidant, the humble chokeberry rates far above blueberries, raspberries, strawberries and blackberries. Fresh berries are best, but dried berries and tea made from the berries are also beneficial.

Anti-inflammatory

The anti-inflammatory properties of chokeberry aid in the prevention of chronic diseases like diabetes, heart disease and problems with the immune system. Chokeberries are noted for strengthening the human immune system by several different processes.

Antiviral activity

One study found that chokeberry was able to inhibit almost 70% of viral plaques from the H1 and H3 flu viruses, and antiviral activity against Influenza type A was also confirmed in another study.

Gastro-protective and antidiabetic effect

Chokeberry juice has been found to reduce injury to the stomach lining due to peptic ulcer. Eating chokeberries also results in improved fasting glucose levels and lipid profiles. Several studies have concluded that they are a good choice in the treatment of diabetes. Anthocyanins found in the fruit also contribute to the prevention of obesity.

Heart Protection

Chokeberry fruit extract has a positive effect on blood pressure, and is recommended as a nutritional supplement to manage hypertension. The berries work as ACE inhibitors, similar to the drug captopril. In one study where subjects took chokeberry supplements for 2 months, 25% of the patients had improvement in blood pressure after one month, and 30% after 2 months.

Prevention of blood clots

Chokeberries help to prevent platelets from clumping together and causing clots. They have also have been found to plaque formation in the aorta and coronary arteries.

Cancer

Studies performed in the laboratory have proven the positive effect of chokeberry on several different cancer cell lines, including breast, leukemia, colon and cervical.

Grow your own!

Ready to claim this plant as your own? Seedlings are available in season at the George O. White Nursery in Licking.

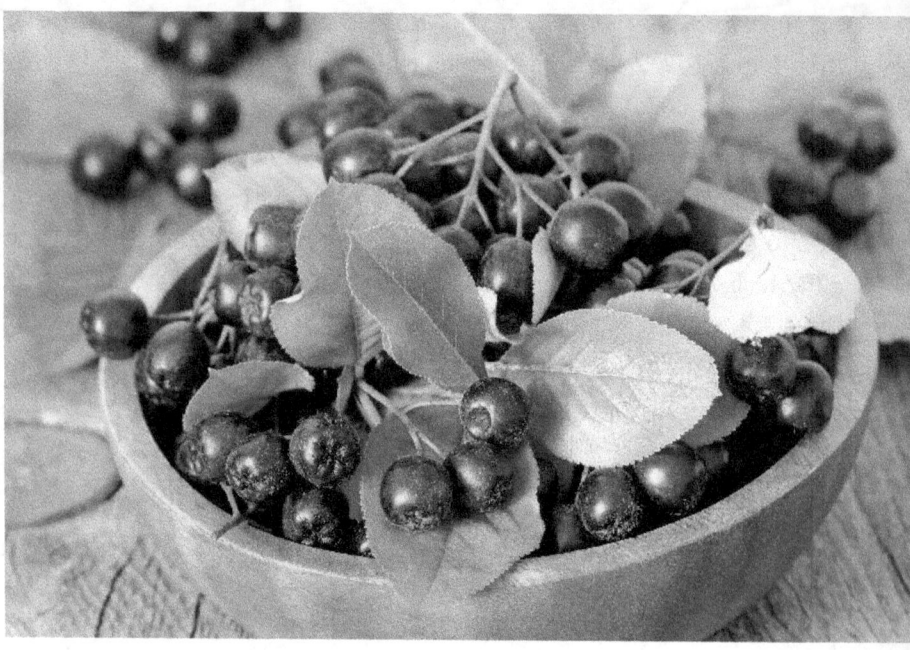

Our native black chokeberry is a super-star in the berry world.

35 LITTLE DIXIE – PASSING ON THE KNOWLEDGE

Since the beginning of time, people have learned to recognize plants and categorize them in three categories: food, medicine, or poison.

Well before Christ walked the earth, ancient societies passed on learned knowledge of plants used to ease pain and treat disease. According to the World Health Organization, 70% of the world's population relies on plants for their primary health care and around 35,000 to 70,000 species have been used as pharmaceuticals, corresponding to 14-28% of the 250,000 plant species around the world having medicinal use. It is presently reported that more than 90 major drugs were discovered by studying traditional herbal use from native plants, but only 17% of plant species have been scientifically investigated for medical potential. One published study showed that Native Americans had 2564 native plants in their arsenal. I personally feel the number is much higher, and there are many, many more remedies yet to be discovered from native plants.

Different areas of the globe have developed their own plant-based medicine systems. It is very interesting that in many cases, different sub-species of the same plant that grow in different areas of the globe have been identified for the same specific use. For example, American licorice (*Glycyrrhiza lepidota*) and Asian licorice (*Glycyrrhiza glabra*) have been used for centuries in the same way for treatment of bronchial asthma in traditional medicine of China and North America.

How do some people, often those who can't read or write, around the world know every plant around them and use them correctly for medicinal purposes? Research has found this knowledge comes from several paths: learning by trial and error, watching how animals use the plants, and passing the knowledge along from generation to generation; a process that seems to be declining in our culture.

In Missouri, one area that has maintained a culture recognizing the value of native plants is Little Dixie, an area consisting of a seven county area that boasts 80 – 90 native plants that are reported to be absent or rarely found in the rest of the state.

Little Dixie

Little Dixie emerged as a cultural region in central Missouri after the War of 1812, and had a distinct identity by the mid 1980's. Populated by migrants from Virginia, Kentucky, Tennessee, North and South Carolina who brought traditions and culture with them (including slaves), today you will find a distinct Southern identity in the local dialect, building design, food, music and even the prominent political party (Democrat).

Justin M. Nolan of the University of Arkansas writes about the Little Dixie region as in the Journal of Anthropology, describing a a community-minded but strongly independent people. One of the ways the community maintains their independence is though regular harvesting of native plants for food, medicine, or pure aesthetics. How has the community gained their formidable knowledge about native plants? According to Nolan, through "family walks outdoors, helping out in the kitchen, and listening to the stories of mothers, fathers, and grandparents."

Depending on the time of year, any one of the 33 main native plants of interest in Little Dixie are gathered from the woods and used to make pies, jellies and jams to be sold or shared with neighbors. In the early spring, it is not uncommon to see local residents picking healthy greens like burdock, lamb's quarters and poke along a country road side; either to be eaten for dinner, or used to make spring tonics and other remedies.

In our own town, the ways of the Amish closely mirror those of the folks from Little Dixie. Both groups, living completely different lifestyles, are proof of the value of our native plants and that traditional knowledge can be passed through the generations.

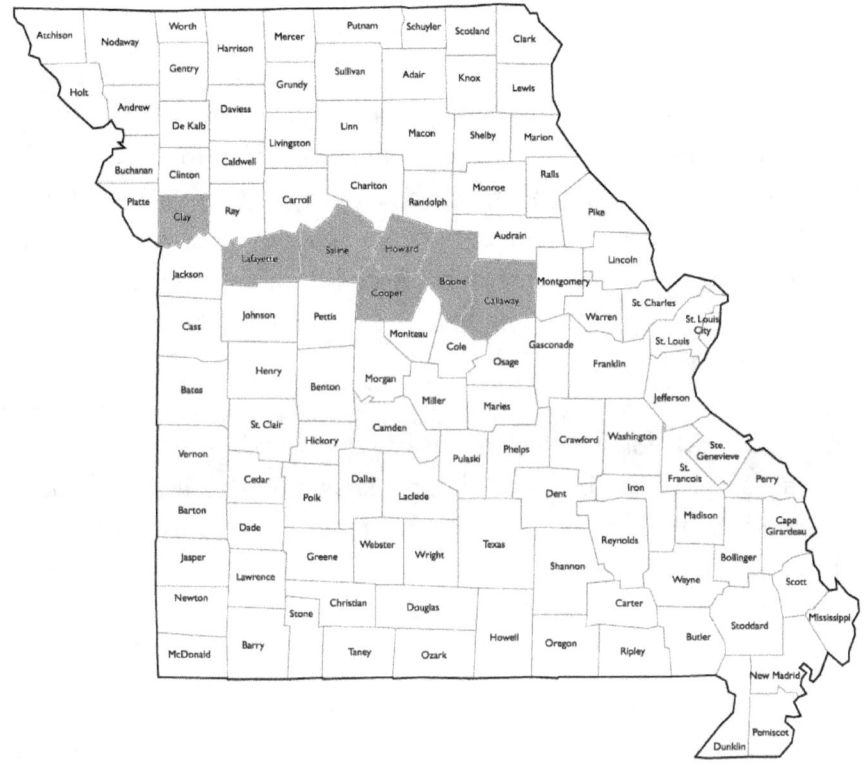

The 7 counties thought to encompass the cultural region known as Little Dixie.

36 THE IMPORTANCE OF TEASELS

Teasels (*Dipsacus fullonum*) have a history of use in textile processing, and dried flower heads from the plant have been used in the past by attaching them to a frame for use as a natural comb to raise the nap and tease the fibers on fabrics, especially wool. Today, metal cards are used for this purpose, but unlike the natural teasel comb, metal can rip the fabric, so teasel frames are still used by natural craftsmen.

Teasels and Lyme Disease

Numerous tick-borne infections cause problems for humans and animals alike. Lyme disease is the best known, but ehrlichiosis, Rocky Mountain spotted fever, and several others also cause problems. Several herbs and their extracts can help to repel several types of ticks with lemon eucalyptus rated the most effective.

When diagnosed with Lyme Disease, we are dealing with a spirochete bacteria from the genus Borrellia. (Spirochetes are also responsible for syphilis). The most common sign of infection is the bullseye rash that occurs the site of a tick bite, about one week later. The rash is not itchy or painful, and up to 50% of infected people never develop a rash. Other early symptoms include fever, headache, and feeling tired. Despite appropriate treatment, about 10 to 20% of people develop joint pains, memory problems, and feel tired for at least six months. Usually, the tick must be attached for 36 to 48 hours before the bacteria can spread, which is why "tick checks' must be done and ticks removed soon after any possible exposure.

While the first line treatment of Lyme Disease is based on antibiotics like doxycycline, chronic Lyme disease results when the body isn't able to clear itself of the infection due to the fact the active bacteria are able to respond to threat (i.e. antibiotics) by changing to a latent form. A small number of plant extracts have been identified to help in this treatment.

Dipsacus fullonum (fuller's teasel) is gaining attention in the treatment of people with Lyme disease, but one has to go deep to locate any clinical trials, as is common for many of the medically active plants. Teasels are possibly the most studied natural cure in the treatment of chronic Lyme disease. One such study was published in 2016 in the Journal of Therapeutic Advances in Infectious Disease. According to the study published in the above journal, over 95% growth inhibition of the bacteria responsible for Lyme Disease was seen with a 2 mg/ml ethyl acetate extraction from the plant, effective on the first day of treatment with greatest effect on day 4, but persistent up until the 8th day of treatment when the study was completed.

In addition to compounds extracted from the plant, teasel seeds contain a low level of crude protein and high level of available lysine – an amino acid that can't be synthesized in the body and has to be obtained from the diet. Lysine has a long history of decreasing herpes simplex cold sore outbreaks and reducing healing time.

It looks like teasels are effective in treating chronic Lyme disease, without the side effects of conventional antibiotics, and less chance of bacterial persistence resulting in a chronic form of the disease.

Cautions

Teasels contain a chemical called dipsacus saponin which is medically important as a procoagulant; that means it helps blood to clot by enhancing platelet function. Typically folks want to stay away from agents that cause clotting, as they can lead to strokes and heart attacks, but there are some conditions that benefit. Dipsacus saponin has many positive health effects, including enhancing memory and learning, and has a protective effect against neurotoxicity from amyloid beta in the brain , a condition that is associated with Alzheimer's Disease.

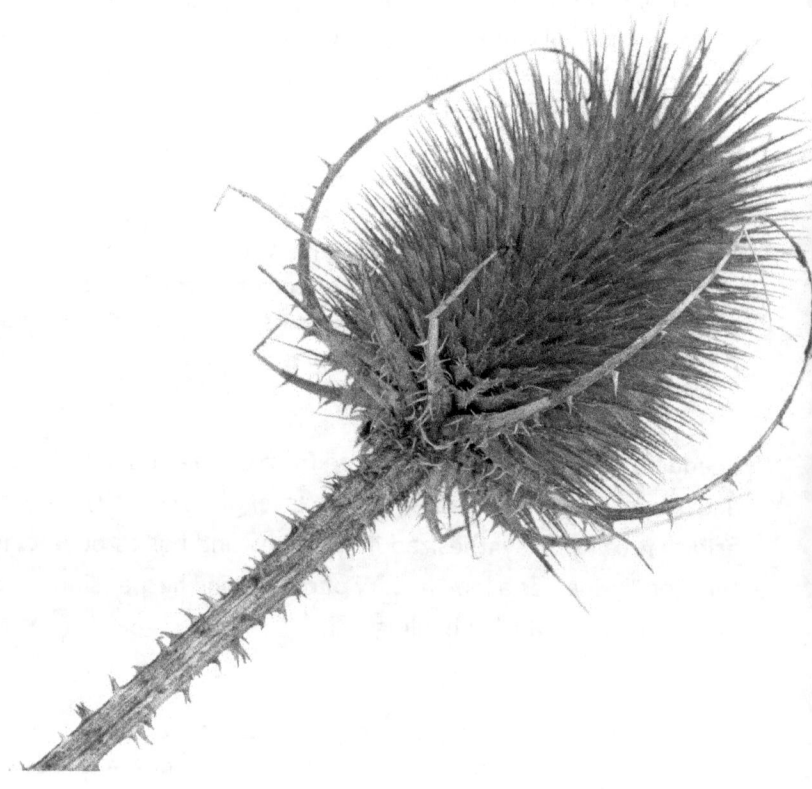

The distinctive Teasel is easily located along roadsides and Missouri ditches.

37 SNAKEROOT

This Mother's Day, I fractured my collarbone after suffering a fall from a horse at a high rate of speed. Despite a complete separation of the bone, I have fully healed in record time, thanks to a poultice containing comfrey, red clover and plantain recommended by Tamara Glascock of *Tamara's Herbes*.

One of the key components of my recovery was a natural tincture for pain and sleep that contains snakeroot, also known as *Rauvolfia serpentine*. The problem with proper bone knitting with a cervical fracture occurs during sleep, as when you turn on your side, typically the bone slides out of proper alignment.

My regimen was as follows: using my trusty coffee grinder, I made a poultice with the above plants, adding a few drops of grape seed oil. At bedtime, I placed the moist poultice directly over the break, covered it with saran wrap, and placed a heating pad. (Note that the common name for comfrey is knit bone, and it surely does!)

Now the hard part: laying flat on my back all night and not disturbing the poultice or the bone alignment. Solution: a nighttime tincture containing snakeroot.

The snakeroot plant is well known to herbalists as a method used to treat insomnia. It has several other uses, including use as a sedative in veterinary medicine. In 1949, German chemists extracted the alkaloid reserpine from snakeroot. Reserpine works by blocking the storage of some of the brain's chemical messengers, including norepinephrine.

Snakeroot is not native to our continent, but is a perennial flowering shrub distributed throughout India. An extremely complex plant, it has over 200 active alkaloids, many of which have medicinal uses, including small amounts of yohimbine, a type of natural viagra.

Blood pressure and anxiety

Reserpine is considered one of the essential 50 fundamental herbs in traditional Chinese medicine, used extensively in the United States from 1954 to 1957 to treat high blood pressure, agitation, epilepsy, and certain mental disorders.

Reserpine helps in sedation and lowering of blood pressure, especially in cases of stress. It works to decrease anxiety by decreasing the amounts of certain chemicals in the brain (e.g. norepinephrine and serotonin), helping to lower blood pressure and decrease anxiety.

Heart arrhythmia

Snakeroot also contains a compound called ajmaline, a first line treatment for ventricular tachycardia, a dangerously fast heart rate originating in the ventricles of the heart. It is so specific to this type of arrhythmia that when given as an intravenous dose it can be used for diagnostic purposes. The blood pressure lowering actions of Reserpine are a result of its ability to deplete chemicals used for transmission of nerve impulses at nerve endings which are normally involved in controlling heart rate, strength of heart contraction and resistance to blood flow.

Snakebite

Like its nickname, Snakeroot has been used as a treatment for snakebite in several regions where it grows naturally. To treat both snakebite and the bites of poisonous insects, the roots and leafbuds are crushed in milk and applied to the area of the bite as a paste.

Nutritional Value

Snakeroot contains high amounts of calcium, zinc, ascorbic acid, riboflavin, thiamin and niacin. Because of the calcium content of the plants, it has been used to aid coagulation, stopping bleeding in the treatment of wounds.

Cautions

Snakeroot should not be used by pregnant women or those with chronic disease of the intestines or stomach, reflux disease, colitis or irritable bowel disease.

38 WILD SWEET POTATO

Wild Parsnips and Sweet Potatoes: good food source with some cautions

Wild sweet potatoes and parsnips grow throughout Missouri. One might be tempted to harvest them as a food source, and they do indeed have nutrients, but preparation is not a casual affair. In the case of wild parsnips, serious skin disorders can be triggered.

Wild Sweet Potatoes (Ipomoea Pandurata) have been a food source in the Ozarks since Native Americans lived on the land. A member of the morning glory family, it is easy to spot with its large white flowers and heart shaped leaves.

Native sweet potatoes cannot be just dug up and eaten like the cultivated variety. Due to the high alkaloid content (that provides medicinal benefits) the large starchy root of the wild sweet potato is bitter, unless cooked in at least two changes of water. Eating the root raw will likely result in vomiting. There are reports of American Indians roasting the root before eating, but pre-soaking the root prior to roasting will lately make it more palatable. The root can also be baked or boiled. The young roots are the best, but are of course smaller. Older roots can grow up to several pounds.

Medicinal Uses

An effective poultice can be made from the root and applied for the pain of painful joints. Root tea has been used as a laxative and diuretic, and as a expectorant for coughs. The tea should be used in only small quantities.

Mole repellant

An infusion made from the water of soaked wild sweet potato can be used to deter moles.

Wild Parsnips

Once considered one of the most important vegetables in our diet, wild parsnips (pastinaca Sativa) are now rarely mentioned. In grandma's day, parsnips were very popular as they are easy to find, can be prepared several ways, and store very well over the winter.

Unlike a lot of wild foods, including the wild sweet potato discussed above, wild parsnips are identical to the cultivated version. (Wild asparagus is also identical to the store-bought version.)

Parsnip is one of the most abundant weeds in the farm country of the Midwest, and if you like them, you shouldn't have to go through the trouble of growing them in your garden. They can be found in loose, agricultural soils, and even along country roads.

It is recommended to harvest parsnips in the fall or early spring when they are at their most nutritious Like many other root vegetables, parsnips contain inulin, a non-digestible starch. During the fall and winter, the plant changes inulin to simple sugars, making the root sweeter, so the later in the fall one harvests the roots, the better as far as the taste.

If you've never tried parsnips, the taste is described as a combination of carrot, banana and apple. They have a strong aroma!

Medicinal Uses

Wild parsnips are mainly used to treat skin inflammations and sores, including psoriasis and vitiligo (loss of skin pigmentation). The active ingredient in the root is xanthotoxin, a compound that can cause severe skin reactions in susceptible people, including photosensitivity, an extreme sensitivity to sunlight.

Plant Identification

It is very important to properly identify wild parsnips, as they resemble water hemlock, a poisonous plant with large roots that look and smell like parsnips.

The thick taproot of the wild parsnip is long and cone shaped. Branching off the root is a light green, hollow stem with deep groves. Leaves are alternate, and branched with saw-toothed edges. Each leaf has 5-15 leaflets. Small, 5-petaled, yellow flowers are arranged in 2-6 inch (5-15 cm) broad umbels at the top of slender stems and branches. Each flat umbel has 15-25 primary rays that contain yellow blossoms. The plant flowers between June-September.

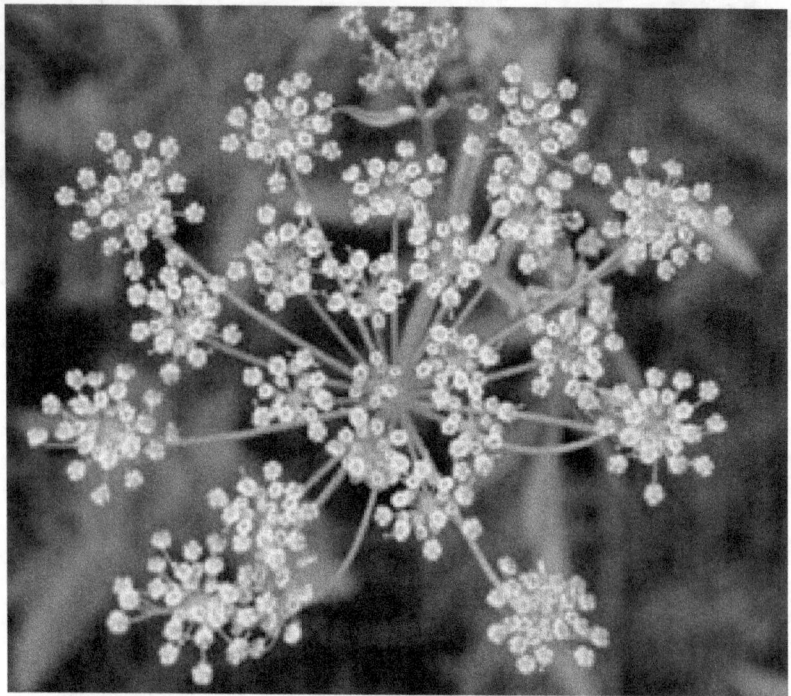

Parsnip in bloom.

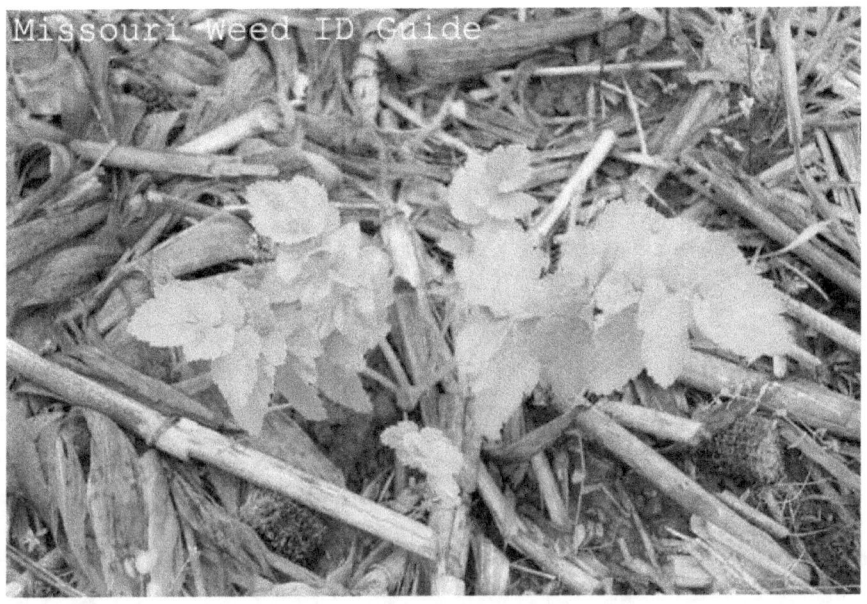

Wild Parsnip: From the University of Missouri Weed ID Guide.

39 ALL SUGARS NOT CREATED EQUAL

Sugar has always been hugely important. Statesman John Adams called molasses "an essential ingredient in American independence." After the Sugar Act of 1764, taxes on sugar products accounted for 97 percent of British revenue. After the 1776 Revolution, the new American government began collecting money from sugar products. Tariffs on imported goods, included sugar constituted the single largest source of federal funds until the institution of income taxes in 1913. During the Civil War, American abolitionists favored beet sugar, because cane sugar was produced with slave labor.

Do you know the difference between cane sugar and beet sugar? There is a world of difference. Almost all sugar comes from 2 sources, non-GMO sugar cane and beet sugar usually made from genetically modified plants. It is important to note that sugar not specifically labeled "cane" is probably made from beets.

Sugar cane is a tropical grass that grows in warm, moist climates. In the United States, sugar cane comes from these four states: Florida, Hawaii, Louisiana and Texas. Sugar cane is a sustainable crop as the only the stems are harvested, leaving the roots to grow again. On the other hand, sugar beets must be planted annually.

When sugar is processed, either from cane or beets, molasses is a by-product. Adding the molasses back to the processed white sugar makes both light brown and dark brown sugars. While white sugar is by law 100% sucrose, brown sugar contains small amounts of potassium, calcium, magnesium and B vitamins. Calorie content is about the same with white sugar having 16 calories per teaspoon compared to 17 calories with brown sugar.

In 2008, the entire sugar beet industry converted to a 100% Round-up ready genetically modified Monsanto product, with no non-GMO alternative. The problem with planting genetically modified plants in the vicinity of their natural counterparts involves inevitable cross-pollination.

In 2005, the major sugar beet seed processors decided to convert the entire US sugar beet production to Roundup Ready genetically modified varieties, developed by Monsanto Company. The industry said farmers needed the genetically modified beets for better weed control. Unlike corn and soybean production where non-GMO alternatives are available, the sugar beet processors did not want that option. The reader is left to decide their reasoning.

Non-corporate sugar beet seed producers in the Willamette Valley in Oregon, where virtually all sugar beet seed is raised, wanted to ensure a 6-mile separation between genetically modified sugar beets and their non-GMO crops. Research shows that is the distance needed to keep GMO contamination around .01%. In addition to contamination of non-GMO crops, farmers are at risk for lawsuits from Monsanto for patent violation if their crops are incidentally contamination with patented Monsanto product. Monsanto files approximately 9 lawsuits a year against farmers who have "improperly used their patented seeds." In the end, only a 3-mile isolation zone was granted, increasing the risk of GMO contamination of conventional and organic seed.

Sugarcane

Sugarcane itself can be eaten as a raw stalk, or more often as a refined sugar. The glycemic index of unrefined sugar cane, the effect it has on blood sugar spikes, is only 43, making it a low glycemic food, especially when compared with the glycemic index of some white breads where the glycemic index is near 100. Unrefined sugarcane has a low glycemic index because sugars derived from plants are processed in your liver, not your small intestine. This means that the sugars from sugarcane -- fructose and glucose -- are more slowly absorbed than sucrose (refined white sugar from any source), decreasing blood sugar level spikes.

Raw sugar

Raw sugar is the residue left after sugarcane has been processed to remove molasses and refine the sugar crystals. While it tastes like brown sugar, it is somewhat different. True raw sugar contains molds and fibers that are considered nutrients, but in order to be sold in the US, raw sugar has to be refined. Types of raw sugar include Demerara sugar, Turbinado sugar, and Barbados sugar.

40 MEDICINAL PLANTS ALONG THE BIG PINEY

Pausing alongside the Big Piney River at the end of Hwy K near Duke, I spotted a two glorious native plants; a bright orange flowered plant, *campsis radicans*, also called Trumpet Vine, and Native Phlox *(paniculata)* with its bright pink flowers. As is common in many riparian plants growing along water, both these beautiful plants have medicinal uses.

Trumpet Vine

Trumpet vine is a native plant that grows in all states east of the Mississippi with exception of Vermont and Maine. It is also found across some of the plains states. A high climbing vine, it produces showy trumpet shaped flowers throughout the summer, and fruit pods that are up to 6 inches long with 2 ridges running lengthwise. It can get out of control and take over, earning the name Hellvine and Devil's shoestring in some areas, but its expansive coverage makes it a good plant for erosion control. The flowers are very attractive to Ruby-throated Hummingbirds, which is not surprising as studies of the trumpet vine reveal five distinct nectary (nectar producing) systems, a phenomenon never before reported among temperate zone plants.

Medicinal Uses

The plant is not considered edible, but has some medicinal uses. The whole dried plant is used to treat yeast infections, and can safely be used as a douche with 4 tablespoons of a tincture made from 1 part plant to 5 parts vinegar, diluted in a pint of warm water.

Cautions

The sap of this plant can cause skin irritation on contact.

Native Phlox

Phlox paniculata is native from New York to Iowa and south to Georgia, Mississippi and Arkansas. In Missouri, it is usually found south of the Missouri River on banks and gravel bars along streams, so my find on the banks of the Big Piney was a perfect habitat. Flowers are aromatic pinkish-purple and sometimes white florets, typically blooming between July and September. Butterflies love the flowers, consisting of a long corolla tube and five flat petal-like lobes. Phlox is also very attractive to hummingbirds.

Medicinal Uses

An extract made from the leaves can be used as a laxative. A poultice made from the leaves has also been used as a drawing solution for boils and as a treatment for eczema.

A tea made from the entire plant has been used to treat stomach and intestinal problems, such as stomachache or indigestion. (Note the laxative effect noted above.)

Phlox flowers are fully edible with a slightly spicy taste. Try a few petals as a beautiful flower garnish on a sald. The flowers can also be crystallized and used as cake and dessert decorations. Only the perennial natives are edible.

If you want to see some magnificent native plants not normally encountered, take a stroll along one of our local rivers, and even creeks. You are sure to find a treasure.

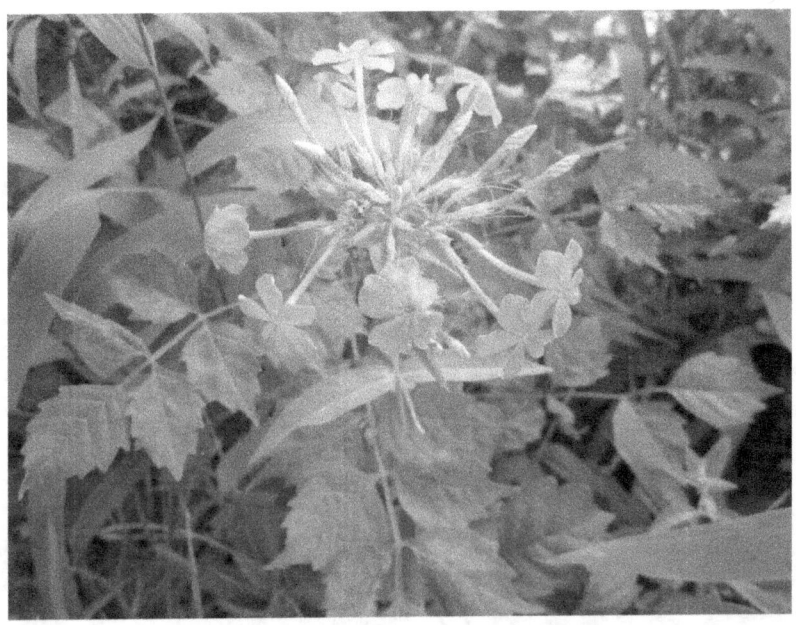

Native phlox in full bloom on the bank of the Big Piney.

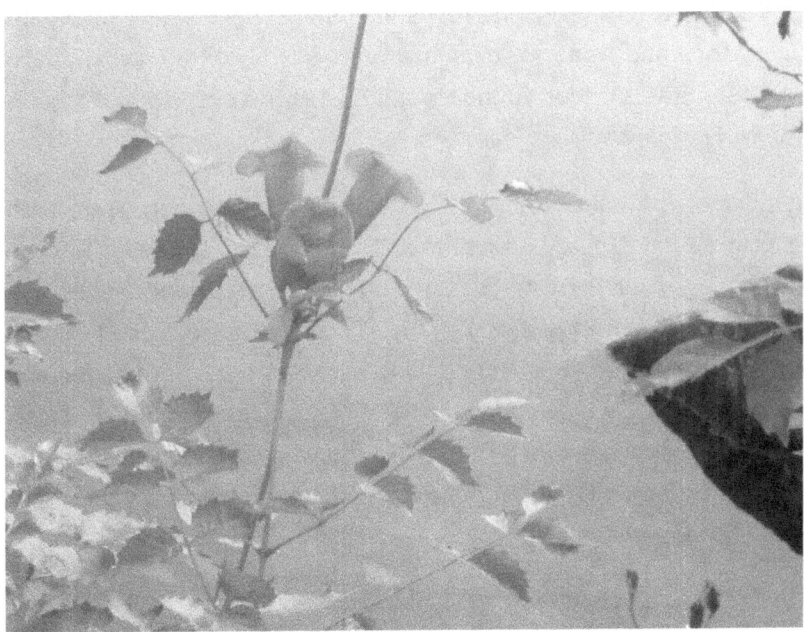

With its brilliant orange blossoms, Trumpet Vine is hard to miss.

41 HOREHOUND – THE FORGOTTEN COUGH REMEDY

Have we reached the point where we have officially forgotten more about natural remedies than the knowledge we still retain? One of the most common questions I hear concerns cough medication for children; what is safe?

One forgotten herb is horehound. Yes, you may occasionally see a package of horehound candy in specialty shops, but since its first documented use during the Roman era, horehound has been used for breathing problems, such as excess mucus production and cough.

The Latin name for horehound, *Marrubium vulgare*, is thought to come from "Mariaurbs," an ancient town in Rome. The plant is native to Europe, Africa and Asia, but over the years has become naturalized in the United States, now found in all states except North Dakota, Louisiana, Florida, and New Hampshire.

A member of the mint family, with a white, woolly, square stem with silver colored hairs, every part of the plant is usable, but generally the leaves are used for their medicinal properties. Horehound leaves feel woolly and are whitish-gray in color. They have an extremely sharp aroma when crushed. Horehound blooms between June and August, with small white flowers that bear burr-like seed pods. Like all mints, the leaves are opposite along the stem. The whole plant is bitter to the taste. It is found in drier, sandy areas. When harvesting, collect right after full flower.

Use in Foods

The leaves can be used to flavor beer and liqueurs. Horehound ale is a fairly common drink in some areas. It is used in a cocktail called Rock and Rye.

As a bitter, it can be used to increase the appetite and aid in digestion. It is an immune booster so drinking a cup of horehound tea once a week can be beneficial.

Medicinal Uses

With Horehound, every part of the plant is usable, and it can be prepared in several ways, the most common being a candy form. Horehound candy is actually a misrepresentation as it is bitter, even with sugar.

While the main use of horehound is to treat coughs, it also has reported used in the treatment of rattlesnake bite when combined with Plantago Lanceolata (Plantain) and applied as a poultice.

Traditional medicine

Celsus, the early Roman medical writer, documented the use of horehound juice as an antiseptic and a treatment for respiratory problems. In veterinary medicine, horehound has been used to treat ulcers, wounds and scabs in animals. Around 150 AD, Galen, "the world's greatest physician," recommended the use of horehound for cough and general respiratory health.
In 1652, a British physician named Nicholas Culpeper wrote, "There is a syrup made of this plant which I would recommend as an excellent help to evacuate tough phlegm and cold rheum from the lungs of aged persons, especially those who are asthmatic and short winded."

Expectorant

Much like the medication Mucinex, Horehound helps to thin secretions to aid in expelling them from the lungs.

Anti-diabetic

The plant has been trialed in the treatment of Type II diabetes. A 2012 study found Marrubiin, one of the primary active compounds found in horehound, to possess "anti-diabetic, anti-atherogenic and anti-inflammatory properties."

Essential Oils

Several recent scientific studies have been conducted on the usefulness of horehound. A 2011 study concluded that the essential oil of M. vulgare (Horehound) contains potent antimicrobial and anticancer properties.

Other Uses

Marrubium vulgare is also used as a natural grasshopper repellent in agriculture.

Homemade Cough Drops

1 cup of crushed horehound leaves
1 cup boiling water
1 cup sugar
1/3 tsp cream of tartar

Put crushed leaves in a measuring cup and cover with boiling water overnight. Pour off liquid into a saucepan, add sugar and cream of tartar and bring to a boil until thickened. Test consistency by checking if it forms into a brittle tread when dropped in ice water. Remove from heat and pour onto waxed paper in teaspoon-sized drops. Let cool.

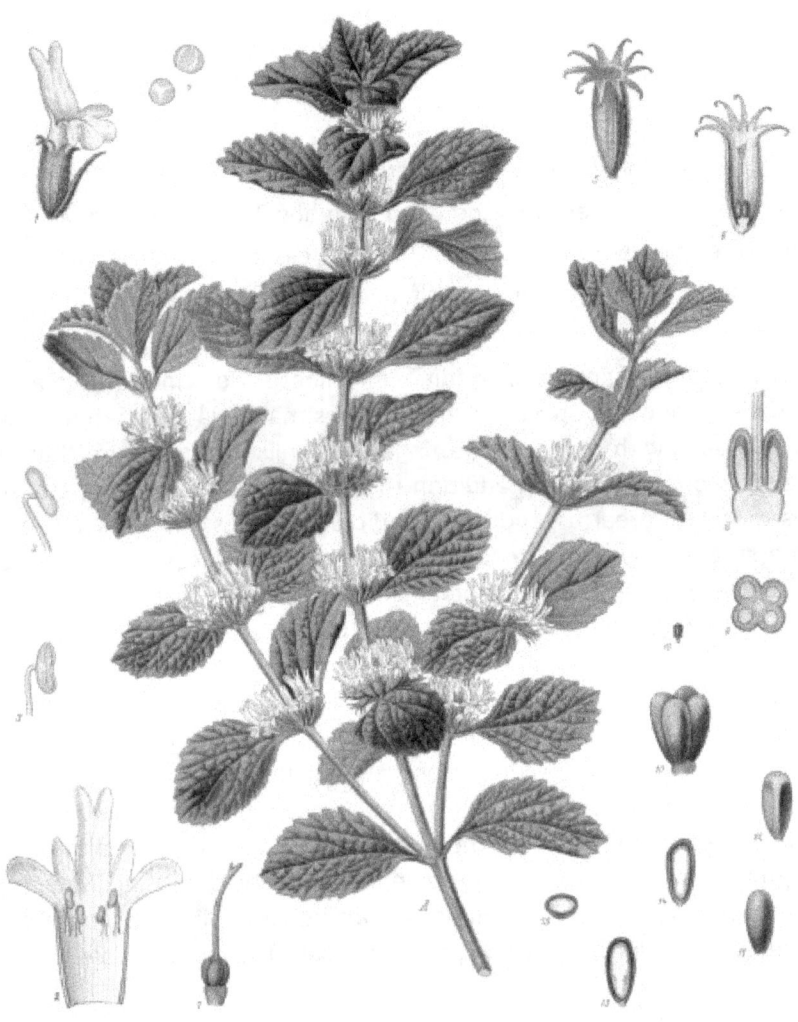

Horehound

42 ACCUPRESSURE FOR DIY, ON THE SPOT HEALING

Out of your blood pressure medication and can't get to the doctor for a day or so? Having anxiety and need help now? Pounding headache and Ibuprofen not working? Why not try acupressure? There are virtually no side effects, you can do it yourself, and relief comes quickly.

Acupressure originated in traditional Chinese Medicine, and is a non-invasive, hands-on approach that involves manipulation of the skin and soft tissues with primarily the fingertips, unlike acupuncture that uses needles on acupoints. In addition to the fingers, other body parts such as knuckles, forearms, and heels, and blunt devices can be used to apply pressure, such as small beads placed at strategic places in the outer ear. Acupressure is easy for anyone to learn and a great thing to have in your arsenal for self-management of pain. It is also FREE.

Acupressure treatment is increasingly being used by health care professionals to treat various types of pain, based on the beliefs of removing obstructions that block energy flow and relieving pain by improving circulation to affected areas. Randomized controlled trials have demonstrated that one month of acupressure treatment can significantly decrease pain, improve function, and decrease disability for at least 6 months. Acupressure has dozens of applications, with blood pressure control, anxiety and pain relief likely the most prevalent.

Headache and other pain

While pain in specific areas of the body has a related pressure point, there is also a universal pressure point for headache and other types of pain. Using your dominant hand, pinch the webbing area between your index finger and thumb of the opposite hand with firm pressure for at least a minute.

For leg pain, place your hand on your calf on the affected side, and slide hand up your leg until your little finger finds a slight depression behind your knee. Apply firm pressure to that area for a least a minute.

Low back pain is a nagging problem for many people. The spasms that come along with the pain are even worse, and often medications are not very effective. If you use a low back support in your chair at work, you are using a form of acupressure. The pressure point for low back pain is located at a region called Ligou LR5 (see photo). It is important to note that the effects of acupressure on low back pain are not only seen in the short term, but have been documented to last up to 6 months.

A very effective treatment to treat lower back spasms is as follows: Lay on your back with legs in the air in the bicycle position, or as high as you can raise them. Making sure your lower back is supported, with your index and middle fingers of each hand, apply pressure to the depression behind each knee for one minute.

Blood Pressure

Acupressure has also been used to effectively lower blood pressure. In addition to using the method described above: putting pressure in the web space between your thumb and index finger; there are two other pressure points recommended. Drawing a line between both ears, find the center point on top of your head, and apply pressure there for at least a minute. Then, using your hands, go to the base of your skull, and find a small depression between your ears and your spine. Using your fingertips, apply pressure to both sides for at least a minute while taking slow deep breaths. I have found this to be very effective.

In one clinical trial involving 80 patients with hypertension, acupressure was applied to the Taichong Accupoint located on the top of the foot, in the depression at the base of the big toe. Blood pressure was checked before, immediately after and at 15 and 30 minutes after intervention. Both systolic and diastolic blood pressure in the experimental group decreased at 0, 15, and 30 min after acupressure with the average following readings: (165.0/96.3, 150.4/92.7, 145.7/90.8, and 142.9/88.6 mmHg).

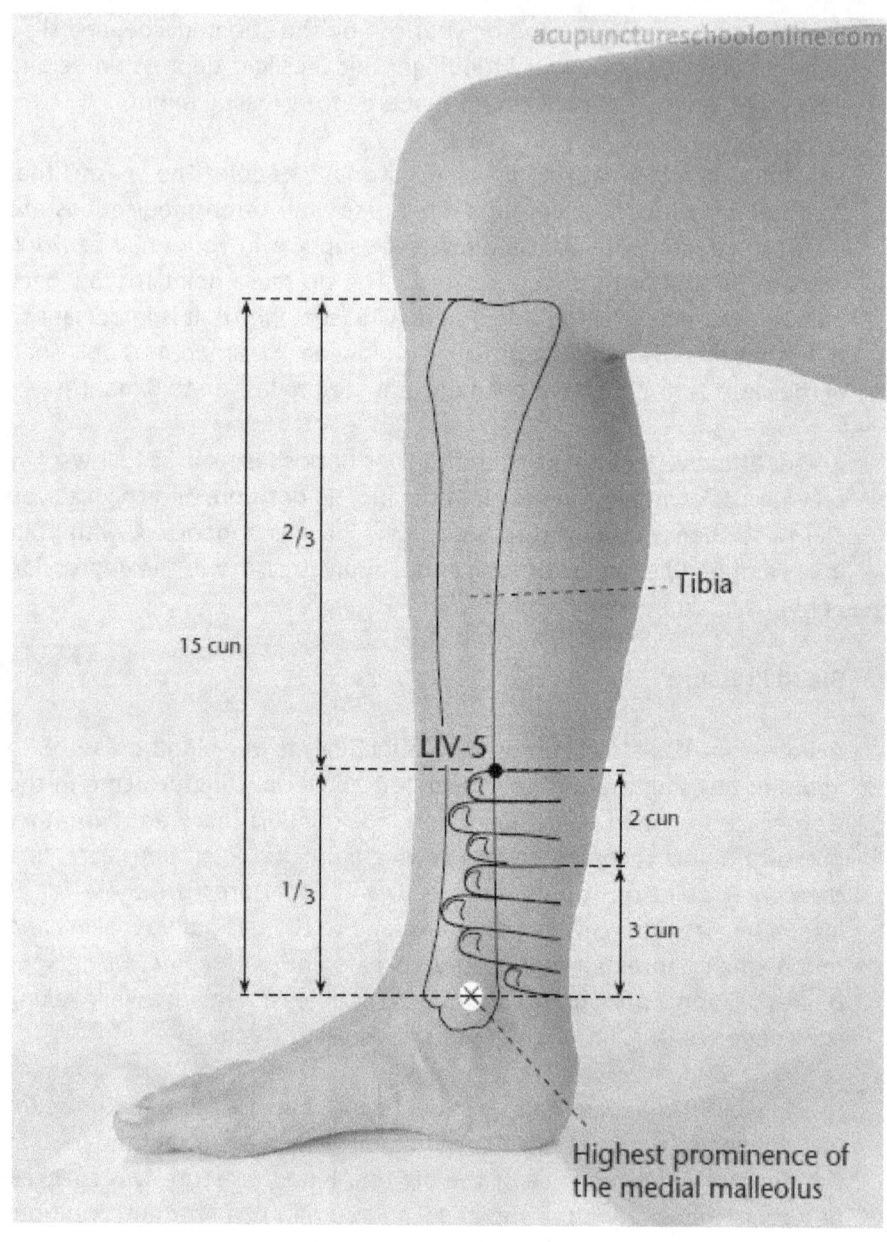

The Ligou LR5 acupressure point. (Photo courtesy of accupunctureschoolonline.com.)

43 ACCUPRESSURE -PART 2

Last week's article discussed the use of acupressure for some types of pain, and also control of blood pressure. It is estimated there are over 400 conditions that benefit from acupressure, with stress and sleep being two of the most common problems addressed.

Stress

A 2006 study involving 76 women who underwent caesarean section, auricular accupressure (in the ear) was studied to see the effect on anxiety, fatigue, and cortisol levels in this group. Elevated cortisol levels in the blood are associated with higher stress levels. Anxiety and fatigue can adversely affect women's postpartum recovery, and typically prescription drugs for these problems are not recommended for women who have just given birth and may be breast-feeding. In addition, elevated cortisol levels can also be passed on in breast milk, and effect on the newborn is unknown.

For the study, women who underwent caesarean section were randomly allocated to two groups: intervention with acupressure, and control with usual care.

The intervention group received auricular acupressure on the shenmen acupoint in the ear (see photo) twice a day (9 AM and 5 PM), and the control group received usual postpartum care. Cortisol levels were drawn, with blood pressure and heart rate recorded. Anxiety and fatigue symptoms were recorded before and after treatment.

Of the 76 women who completed the study, those who received auricular acupressure had significantly lower cortisol levels, heart rate, anxiety symptoms, and fatigue symptoms than women in the control group who did not receive acupressure at 5 days postpartum. The researchers concluded that auricular acupressure is an effective non-pharmacological method for reducing cortisol levels, heart rate, anxiety, and fatigue in early postpartum after caesarean section.

A similar study was used to treat elderly patients with acute hip fracture who were being transported by ambulance. 38 patients were divided into 2 groups. One group received auricular acupressure for hip pain, and the other group received acupressure at "sham," or non-active acupressure points in the ear. Baseline demographic information, anxiety level, pain level, blood pressure, and heart rate were obtained before the administration of the appropriate acupressure intervention. The level of anxiety, level of pain, hemodynamic profiles, and level of satisfaction were reassessed once the patients arrived at the hospital. Patients in the true intervention groups had less pain and lower heart rate on arrival at the hospital than did patients in the sham control group. As a result, the patients in the true intervention group reported higher satisfaction in the care they received during the ride to the hospital.

Sleep

Poor sleep quality is a problem faced by millions. With side effects seen from pharmaceutical sleep aids, there an increasing interest in alternative treatments. A review of thirty-two major studies looking at the effects of acupressure on sleep quality as compared with standard treatments showed that even fragile populations such as the elderly and dialysis patients can benefit from acupressure. Standardized treatment protocols involved pressure for one to five minutes per acupoint, delivered three to seven times a week for three to four weeks with the HT7 (Shenmen)wrist acupoint used in most procedures (see photo).

In another study testing the effect of acupressure on sleep in older women, four pressure points were chosen, with treatments carried out for 4 weeks with the same time length and technique in both the acupressure and non-acupressure groups. The intervention time was limited to 10 minutes. It was done 1 to 2 hours before sleeping, each night (except Fridays) by circular pressure massage covering 1 cm diameter. It was concluded that acupressure alone can improve sleep quality at a rate of 22% in menopausal women by massage on the effective points. Researchers suggest that acupressure may have an important role in managing sleep disturbances and improve sleep quality in women with menopause, and can be used as a self-care method for sleep disorders.

Summary

This is a very brief review. There are hundreds of indications for acupressure, with more in the process of being added.

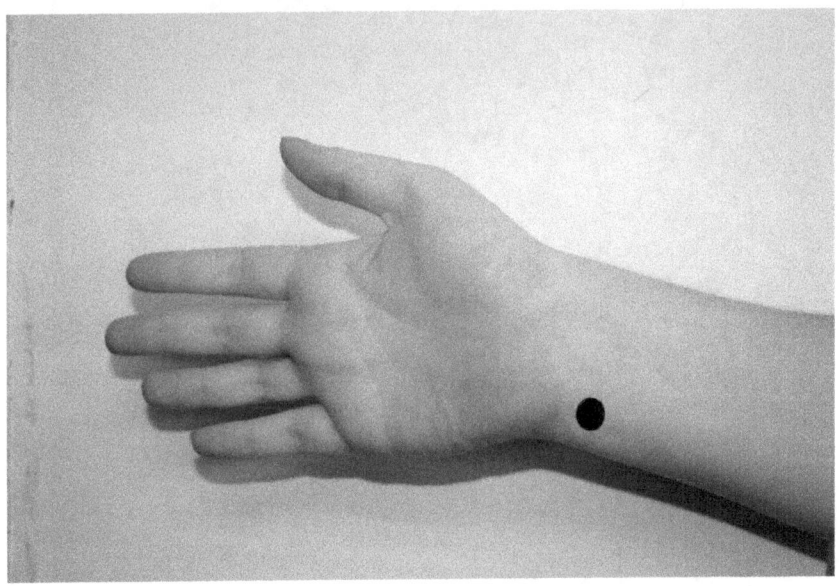

HT7 wrist acupoint

Marie Lasater

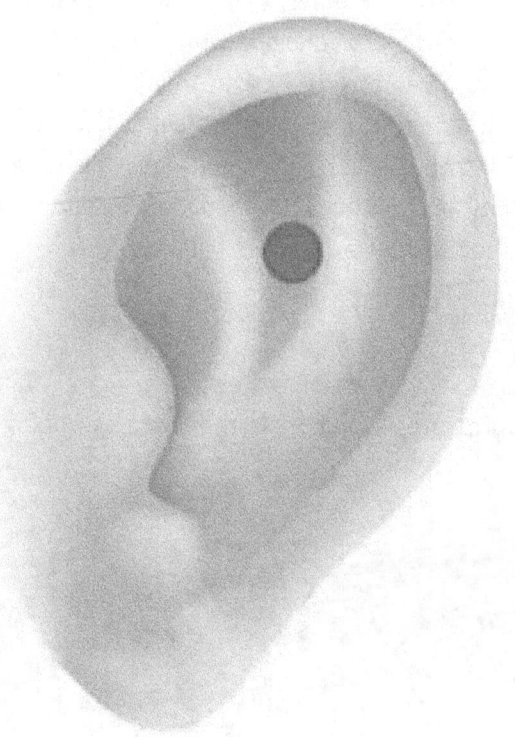

Shenmen accupoint in the ear

44 NEEM: HERBAL POWERHOUSE

I first encountered an extract called Neem, made from the *azadirachta indica* plant several years ago. It was recommended to me to treat the skin and coat of a black German Shepherd who had repeated skin conditions due to fungus. In addition to being an excellent antifungal, Neem is known for a wide range of medicinal properties. Different parts of the Neem tree, including its fruit, seed, bark, leaves, and root have been shown to possess antiseptic, antiviral, antipyretic, anti-inflammatory, anti-ulcer, antimalarial, antifungal and anticancer activity.

Most products are made from the leaves, but Neem seeds are the main source of Neem oil and Azadirachtin, the main active ingredient. A single tree can produce almost 50 pounds of fruit per year. The Neem tree is native to India, where 60% of the estimated 25 million Neem trees are located, and loves growing in a tropical to subtropical climate. It thrives in hot weather, but it can handle the occasional cold spell down to about 35 degrees F. It can be successfully grown in Missouri, but has to be kept in a pot and brought inside during the winter.

Nutrition

Neem leaves themselves are 23% carbohydrate, 7% protein, and are rich in amino acids and calcium. They are safe to eat, and serve as an anti-helmintic (wormer).

Cancer

Active components in Neem have been shown to have anti-cancer and anti-cancer activity. Nimbolide, an ingredient found in the leaf, stops tumor growth and induces apoptosis (cancer cell death). This effect has been confirmed in several studies looking at the effect of Neem on cervical cancer, breast cancer, colon cancer, prostate cancer, lymphoma, leukemia and liver cancer.

Liver Protection

A water extract made from the leaves of the Neem tree has been shown to protect the liver against toxic agents, including drugs that harm the liver. Tylenol is a drug that is very toxic to the liver.

Wound healing and anti-ulcer

Neem has been used for thousands in years in India to treat stomach ulcers. A poultice made of Neem leaves applied to wounds promotes new blood vessels, bringing oxygen and promoting wound healing.

Diabetes

Rutin and quercetin found in Neem leaves significantly lower glucose levels in the blood, and have been found to be an effective strategy to lower blood sugar levels after eating a meal.

Antimicrobial

Neem is an effective antifungal, antiviral and antibacterial agent. It is effective against food-borne pathogens, and also valuable as a mouth rinse as it kills Streptococcus mutans, the bacteria that cause cavities. Neem twigs are used to clean the teeth in some third world countries.

Neem leaves can also be used to maintain the quality of preserved meat. When used against viruses, Neem extract has been shown to inhibit the poliovirus and the coxsackie virus. Neem leaf paste is used to treat fungal infections on the skin of animals. A water extract of Neem is also effective against aspergilla.

Use as pesticide

Neem is especially useful as a safe pesticide, and is considered a "green approach." Farmers in other countries use it on their crops, and it has been shown to prevent blue tongue virus outbreaks in cattle. Neem is used for mosquito control, and is also effective against the pulse beetle. Neem oil at a concentration of 10ml/kg prevented egg laying, reduced population buildup of beetles and minimized seed damage as compared to common pesticides. It is likely Neem oil is also effective against the Japanese beetle that plagues us every year from May to the end of July, but there are no published studies.

45 ROSE HIPS: PACKED WITH NUTRITION AND SO MUCH MORE

Rose hips are the fruit of the rose bush. They are super-packed with essential nutrients that often go to waste. Among the nutrients found in rose hips are vitamins A, C, and E, plus minerals calcium, magnesium, potassium, selenium, manganese and sulfur. Although rose allergies exist, no other side effect from the use of rose hips has been documented. Many popular over the counter vitamins contain rose hips as a terrific source of Vitamin C.

Rose hips mature on the rose bush in late summer or early autumn, and ripen about four months after they first appear. When ripe, they are firm and plump. To harvest, pick or cut them from the bush. Obviously, don't use rose hips from bushes that have been treated with chemical pesticides. If you want to save the seeds to grow new rose bushes, cut open the fruit and scrape out the seed. You can also blend a cup of rose hips in a blender with a cup of water. The nicks the seeds attain during the process help them to germinate when processed. Pour the seed mixture through a strainer, then spread the wet seeds on a paper towel or newspaper to dry. This method can be used to harvest many types of tiny seeds. To germinate rose seeds, cold stratification is required. This can be accomplished by placing the seeds in a plastic bag filled with moist peat moss or coffee grounds in your refrigerator for about 2 months. The dreaded multiflora rose also produces rose hips with all the benefits they offer, but please don't plant multiflora rose!

As a Food

Foods prepared with rose hips are considered a delicacy throughout the world. Unfortunately, in the United States they generally go to the compost pile. Most rose hips have a sweet, tangy flavor. You can make a tea by steeping the chopped hips in hot water. Homemade tea will have to be strained to remove the hairy seeds, but commercially available tea has been more highly processed. Rose hips are easily dried by using a dehydrator, or simply laying them out on the counter. They can then be stored for later use.

There are many uses for rose hips in syrups, jams and jellies. To make jelly or syrup, first boil the hips to extract the juice and sweeten with sugar or honey for syrup. Add pectin to make jelly. In Sweden, rose hips are used to prepare 'Nypon soppa,' a traditional Swedish fruit soup. In Turkey, rose hips are used to make a fruit juice, and a popular probiotic dairy product called Rosalact is fortified with rose hips and licorice extract. It is safe to say that rose hips have been largely neglected in North America.

There is a lot of current research into the use of rose hips in order to improve the stability and shelf life of some foods. Among the uses are as a partial substitute for sodium nitrate in pork hotdogs. This is important since it means that the concentration of this poorly tolerated additive could be decreased in some of our food products.

Next Week: Medicinal Uses of Rose Hips.

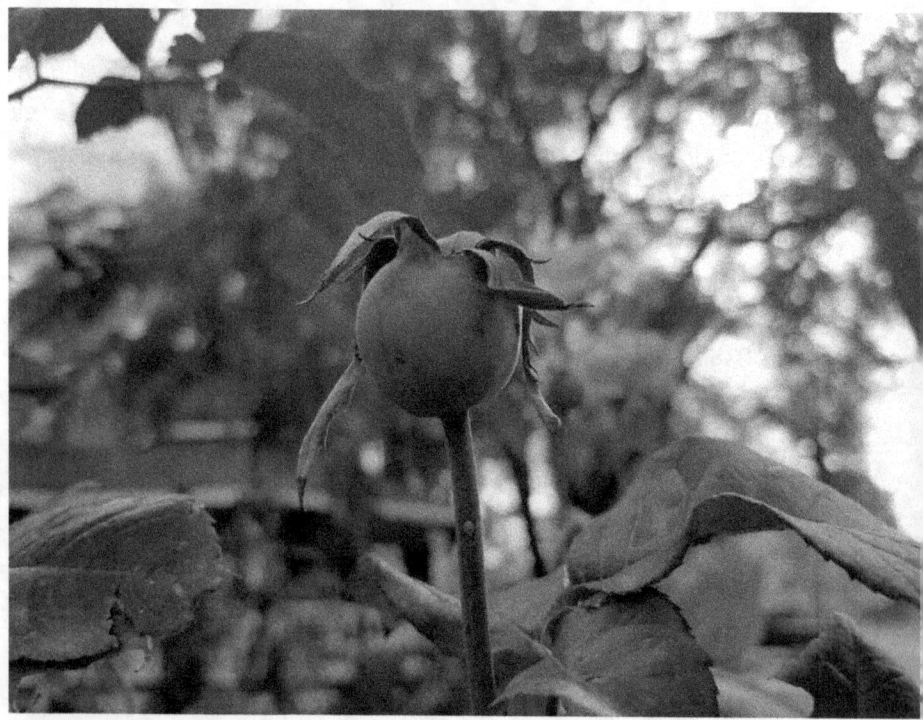

A mature rose hip in a Texas County garden. *Photo courtesy of Mike Baker*

46 ROSE HIPS – PART 2

In last week's column we discussed the nutritional properties of rose hips, but the often discarded fruit of the rose bush has so much more to offer in the way of natural healing.

Medicinal Uses

Rose hip extracts have been proven to help the following conditions: non-alcoholic fatty liver disease, osteoarthritis, rheumatoid arthritis, obesity, cancer, kidney stones, depression, and skin issues. There are multiple rose hip pharmaceutical products on the market.

Cardiac Protection

In a study involving 31 obese subjects, 40 grams of rose hip power were taken daily over 6 weeks. Compared to a control group who did not receive rose hips, the treated individuals saw a significant decrease in systolic (the top number) blood pressure and total cholesterol. Investigators concluded that daily consumption of rose hip power has the ability to significantly protect the heart by lowering blood pressure and cholesterol.

Cancer

The anticancer properties of rose hips have been evaluated in various cancer cell lines, including cervix, non-small cell lung cancer, colon cancer, liver cancer, and prostate cancer. All groups found significant decreases in cancer cells after incubating these cancer cell lines with whole rose hip extract or its purified fractions.

Arthritis

Rose hip powder has been shown to reduce symptoms associated with rheumatoid inflammation in clinical trials. The powder works by delivering anti-inflammatory molecules, and lowering the levels of C-reactive protein (CRP), a protein produced in the liver in response to inflammation. If you suffer with arthritis, your blood work will include testing for C-reactive protein, enabling your physician to easily evaluate the effect rose hips have in treating your condition.

Obesity

Rose hips have been found to have a role in obesity prevention. Scientists delving into the effect of rose hips on obesity found they prevented lipid deposits in fat cells, leading to a decrease in body weight. A study was conducted on volunteers who took a daily supplement of rose hip extract and found that this supplementation contributed to reducing the levels of abdominal fat without any undesirable side effects. The researchers confirmed the previous findings in animal models and proposed rose hips as "a promising candidate for anti-obese therapies."

Kidney stones

Calcium oxalate kidney stones are the bane of many folk's existence. If you haven't passed one of these stones yourself, chances are you know someone who did. Currently, there is an important lack of drugs for their prevention and treatment. In animals treated with rose hips, researchers observed a decrease in calcium oxalate content in treated rats as well as a drop in number of calcium oxalate kidney stones.

Alzheimer's

At this time, rose hips from the Damask rose are one of the most promising medicinal plants for Alzheimer treatment. In animal studies, extract from the rose hips of this particular rose

found an improvement in spatial and long-term memory. The effects are likely due to the prevention of development of amyloid in the brain, a type of sticky substance that prevents brain synapses from working properly.

Anxiety and Depression

Aromatherapy with rose hip extract has been proposed as an alternative therapy for the management of psychiatric disorders, including anxiety or depression. Benefits of aromatherapy are due to the chemical composition of essential oils, which contain active compounds capable of stimulating different central nerve system areas. This stimulation leads to a release of neurotransmitters, for example serotonin, responsible for relaxing effects.

Skin Problems

Oil extracted from rose hip seeds has huge popularity as an anti-aging skin care product. It helps to remove age spots, reduce scars, treat acne and decrease wrinkling of the skin.

One of the most common skin disorders is atopic dermatitis, a chronic inflammatory disorder

that mainly affects children. Treatments for skin lesions associated with this disease are focused on a suppressed inflammatory response, but most therapies are just temporary because of the side effects associated to long time exposure to steroid treatments. It has long been recognized that to improve the quality-of-life for thousands of infants worldwide, new drugs to treat atopic dermatitis are needed in order to solve the problem without potential dangerous effects.

Topical application of extracts from multiflora rose root extracts improved atopic dermatitis in test animals. The effect seems to be related to the anti-inflammatory properties of multiflora rose.

47 COMMON LOUSEWORT

A plant we don't hear much about, but native to the southeastern part of the Ozarks, is Lousewort; Latin name Pedicularis canadensis. The plant in itself is beautiful, with twisting pink to purple flowers when it blooms between April and May. It has the interesting peculiarity of being parasitic on the roots of other plants, so if you attempt to grow it yourself, rather than finding it in the wild, be careful where you plant it, as it can potentially pick up toxic components of other plants through its roots. In addition to its taproot, Lousewort sends out side roots that can attach to the roots of nearby plants such as grasses and tap nourishment from them. It can grow successfully without host plants, however.

Look for Lousewort in dry and open woodlands, prairies, shaded glades, bottomlands, alongside streams and in wooded valleys; usually in acidic soils. It often grows in large colonies.

Medicinal Uses

When used in medicine, Lousewort is most known as a skeletal muscle relaxant. As opposed to smooth muscles, like your intestines, skeletal muscles are those you can move at will, and often cause pain and discomfort. While not a pain medicine, anyone who has had a major injury can likely appreciate how helpful non-narcotic muscle relaxers are in easing pain. A lot of pain is based in the skeletal muscles of the neck and shoulders, and Lousewort is helpful in relaxing these muscles. Side note: many headaches are due to posture and tension in neck muscles, so lousewort may be helpful in treating headaches of this nature.

Other uses for Lousewort in traditional medicine include antioxidant, stimulation of the immune system, anti-diabetic, antibacterial, antifungal, antitumor, protection of the brain and liver, diuretic, fever reducer, blood thinner and DNA-repairing properties.

Herbal Combinations

Lousewort can be combined with other plants to boost its healing properties. Black Cohosh and Skullcap also have muscle relaxant effects. By adding a strong anti-inflammatory like arnica, willow bark or turmeric, you can make a potent tincture to treat pain and inflammation.

Medicine Preparation

The best time to make a tincture with Lousewort is when the plant is in flower, usually in April or May. Chop the leaves, and put 1 part plant and to 2 parts ethanol.

Dosage

According to the literature, side effects are few, but some people experience "feeling spacey" with the tincture. Onset of action is rapid, and it is recommended to initially take 3 – 4 drops under the tongue or in a glass of water, then wait about 10 minutes and repeat the dose if necessary. After your own effective dose is established, repeat the dose whenever you feel pain returning.

Safety

Another advantage of Lousewort is its general good safety record; negative side effects are uncommon. The most common is mild disorientation. For some people this will be enough to warrant trying a different remedy, for others it can be helpful as it further reduces their sensation of pain.

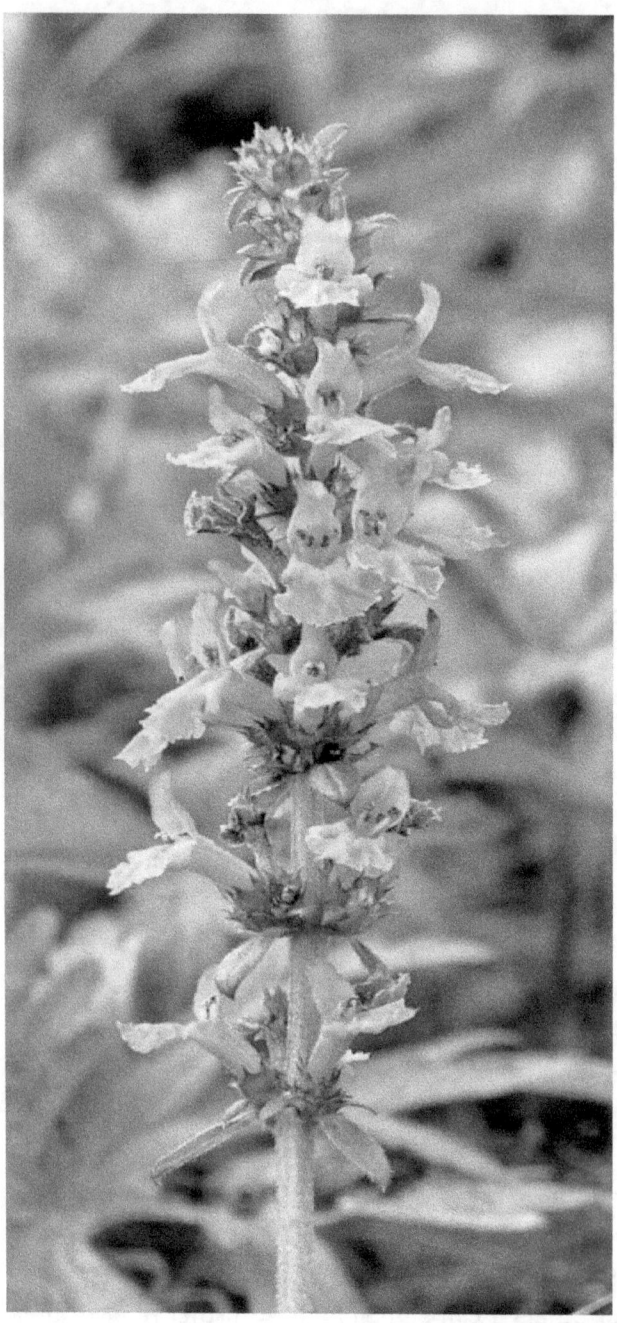

Lousewort has beautiful twisting pink to purple flowers when it blooms between April and May.

48 REVISITING FLUORIDATON AFTER PASSAGE OF THE FLUORIDE PROTECTION BILL

It's been a year and a half since I drove to Jefferson City and testified to the Senate regarding HB1717, The fluoride protection bill. It didn't go well. Despite my attempts to educate the Senators, including emails and trips to their offices, they remained incredibly misinformed about the bill. In addition, three lawyers from the DNR were permitted at the meeting; rudely laughing and disrupting my allotted 3 minutes to speak.

At first glance it would appear that the Department of Natural Resources would attempt to keep industrial-grade fluoride chemicals -- typically hydrofluorosilicic acid or and sodium silicofluoride – out of our water supply, but they are complicit in preventing their removal from the public water. The fluoride protection bill requires 90 days notification to the DNR prior to even a VOTE to remove fluoride from the water. I know firsthand the resources they can throw at the issue to ensure a vote doesn't come to pass.

HB1717 not only passed fluoride protection, but in the 11th hour a separate item was added on one day, voted on the next day (ONE DAY PRIOR TO END OF SESSION) no public notice, no public comment period, nothing. Guess what was tacked onto the bill? DNR Multipurpose Water Resource Program Fund adding 3 new DNR jobs at taxpayer expense of $220K a year. Also, despite prior removal of the emergency clause, Rep. Sonya Murray Anderson helped to get the emergency clause added back into the bill, meaning that the bill was enacted immediately upon signing, rather than after the first of the year as is common with most bills. Why is preventing removal of fluoride from the water an emergency? There is no such urgency if a community wanted to add fluoride to the water, which no community wants to do, unless mandated by law, as is the case in Arkansas. Representatives that should be commended for voting NO on the bill include Robert Ross, Mike Moon and Will Kraus.

Eureka Springs, Arkansas has seen rising lead levels after fluoride was added to their water supply following two public votes AGAINST fluoridation. Fluoride causes lead to leach from pipes and brass fittings. In an article published in February this year by Becky Gillette of the *Eureka Springs Independent,* Sen. Bryan King of Green Forest, Arkansas advised voters interested in reversing the decision about fluoridation of public water supplies to contact members of the Arkansas Senate City County Local Committee to express support for local control, without interference by the state. (Fluoridation of water at Carroll Boone Water District began in July 2015 as a result of a mandate by the state legislature that all public water systems with more than 5,000 customers fluoridate drinking water supplies.)

Prior to HB171 being passed, it was a simple matter to remove fluoride from the municipal water supply, requiring a simple vote by the City Council. After agreement by city Council members, fluoride could then be removed immediately. Since passage of the bill, no towns in Missouri have been able to successfully remove fluoride from their water, with Warsaw and Sullivan as the last two towns able to get fluoride removed from their drinking water. Interestingly, Sen. Dave Schatz, who hails from Sullivan, voted FOR the fluoride protection bill, but now benefits from removal of fluoride in his hometown.

List of towns in Missouri that successfully removed Fluoride since 2010 prior to passage of the Fluoride Protection Bill in March, 2016 in Missouri:

10/5/2010: O'Fallon

2/7/2012: Bolivar

5/1/2012 Pevely

2/22/2013: Smithville

5/12/2014: Buffalo

8/21/2014: Waynesville

8/8/2015: Carl Junction

8/15/2015: Warsaw

5/19/2015: Sullivan

Addendum: List of towns in Missouri that have removed Fluoride after passage of the 2016 Fluoride Protection Bill:

November 2018: Houston

49 MAKING HERBAL TINCTURES

By: Tamara Glascock

When using herbs for their medicinal properties, there are several ways that they can be prepared. Teas, tinctures and extracts are the fastest, most efficient way to introduce herbs into your system. The first step in creating your own herbal medicine is understanding the difference between teas, tinctures and extracts.

Teas are created using water, and are the most efficient, potent and reliable forms of herbal medicine. Teas alone cannot be used for long-term preservation of herbal properties, but they are wonderful when you need fast relief.

Tinctures and extracts are often used interchangeably. Both are created using alcohol as a menstruum to capture the healing properties of the herb. The difference is in the amount of herb used in proportion to alcohol. They have a shelf-life of several years. Both deliver relief as quickly as teas. The only drawback is that they take a bit longer to make than tea.

When making your own tinctures, you must know the herb you are working with. Some medicinal properties are best extracted using water, while others are best extracted using alcohol. Each liquid will extract different properties from the plant. When making tinctures, the simplest solution is to make a water/alcohol solution, which is called an extract.

Start by gathering your herbs

You will want to gather enough of the plant material to fill ¾ of a quart-size mason jar. Choose healthy, clean plants at their peak. For above-ground parts (leaves, flowers, seeds), harvest while the plant is in bloom, usually in the spring/early summer. Some wonderful plants to turn into tinctures during this time of year are chickweed, plantain leaf, and dandelion leaf.

After harvesting the aerial parts of a plant for tincturing, lightly shake the plant to detach any loose insects, dirt or debris. To process your plant material, rinse it under a gentle spray of water, if desired. Using sharp scissors or knife, cut your plant material into smaller pieces. There is no exact size here. I like to cut them into 1" size pieces. This is an easily workable size for me and allows room in my jar for plenty of liquid. Using a blunt object like the fat end of a knife, or a pestle, bruise the leaves so that they begin the process of releasing their medicinal components.

For roots, wait until the plant is finished blooming and begins to die off. This is usually in the fall/early winter. Some useful roots to tincture at this time of year are burdock, yellow dock, and dandelion root. You want to select roots that are firm and moist. I prefer to harvest roots early in the morning, just after sunrise. Tap as much dirt and debris from the roots as you can. Using a soft-bristled toothbrush, very gently scrub any remaining dirt and rocks from roots under cool water. To process, use sharp pruning shears or knife to cut roots into small pieces. The smaller, the better when working with roots.

Choose your menstruum

When making tinctures, I prefer the use of Everclear, but vodka is a sufficient substitute if necessary. Add enough alcohol to fill the jar to the bottom of the rim. Use a butter knife to remove as much air from the jar as possible. Cap tightly and give the jar a good shake. Add more alcohol, if necessary. Label your jar with the date and contents, and store it in a cool, dark place for 3-6 weeks, shaking vigorously once a day. The longer you allow it to sit, the more potent your extract will be.

Now, we wait.

50 TINCTURES ~ PART 2

By: Tamara Glascock

Your tincture has been extracting for a few weeks, right? Now it is time to strain out the solid plant material from the alcohol. Gather up something to strain with. I prefer to use a small stainless steel kitchen strainer, followed by a piece of cheesecloth or thin cotton material in order to get all of the fine bits. This is not absolutely necessary, but gives a prettier final product. Small leftover bits of plant matter will not affect the shelf-life or efficacy of the finished extract.

Strain the tincture, but do not dispose of the plant matter. Set this aside.

Measure out the amount of alcohol tincture you have, then place it in a sealed glass container.

In a heat-safe glass jar, measure out twice the amount of distilled water as you have of the alcohol tincture. For example, if you have 16 ounces of alcohol tincture, you will need 32 ounces of distilled water.

Place your leftover plant material from the alcohol tincture into the distilled water. If desired, add in a bit of fresh plant material.

Place the glass vessel you are using in a pot of water over low to medium heat and allow to brew for 3-6 hours. This is the tricky part. You do not want this to get hot enough to evaporate off all of the medicinal properties of the herbs, but you want it hot enough to extract them. If you see a small amount of steam rising gently from the tea, this is perfect. If you see steam rolling off the tea as it brews, you are running too hot and need to lower your temperature.

When your tea has steeped for the desired amount of time strain the plant material from the tea. You can now dispose of the plant material. Place the tea back over low to medium heat and allow to remain there until your tea has reduced by half. For example, if you have 20 ounces of tea after straining out the plant matter, allow it to cook until you only have 10 ounces remaining. This may take several hours, or possibly even a full day, depending on the amount you are working with. This is a concentrated tea.

When your tea is reduced to the proper amount, mix the alcohol tincture with the tea. You now have a potent medicinal extract. Label it clearly with the date, the plant material used, and the type of alcohol used. Store your extract in a cool dark place. This should keep for many years without losing potency when stored properly.

To use your extract, the dosage will be dependent on the herb, as well as the healing benefit you are hoping to achieve. It is important to be familiar with the herbs you are working with, as well as any possible side effects.

Extracts can be taken orally or used topically. Many people find extracts are easier to take orally when added to a small amount of water or juice. To use topically, they can be applied directly to the skin, or diluted with water and used as a wash.

51 WHO LET THE BEETLES OUT?

The Asian Lady beetles, who are no ladies at all, love to bite, crawl in your clothes and invade your house. Where did they come from? Well, the USDA, Forestry Service and state and private agencies have released them on purpose. During the 1960s to 1990s, the U.S. Department of Agriculture attempted to establish the Asian lady beetle to control agricultural pests, especially of pecans and soybeans, releasing them as a biological control agent. The beetles are voracious feeders with adults capable of eating 15 to 65 aphids per day and each larva eating 90 to 370 aphids during its development. As they have been fairly recently introduced to the United States, they have no natural enemies.

In a 2003 article by Daniel A. Suomi, PhD entitled "Good Bug Gone Bad or Biocontrol Gets a Black Eye," he describes residents complaining about ladybugs everywhere, including waking them from sleep with the bugs crawling over their face. This happened at my house when an Asian Lady Beetle crawled into my son's ear, causing quite a bit of damage.

The beetle we are currently dealing with is the multicolored Asian lady beetle, Harmonia axyridis, a native of Japan, Korea, and other parts of Asia. As Dr. Suomi reports, numerous releases of the beetle have occurred throughout the United States including Georgia, South Carolina, Louisiana, Mississippi, Missouri, California, Washington, Pennsylvania, Connecticut and Maryland. From my memory, I recall a news report of an Asian beetle release in mid 2003, imploring people not to kill the beetles, but rather vacuum them up and release them.

In their natural habitat, the beetles cluster together in the winter months to stay warm, usually on the sides of cliffs. Guess what? Your house is a substitute for that cliff, and they love light colored walls with a southwest exposure. They are usually at their worst in October and November, because that is when they hibernate.

Unlike our native species, this "ladybug" can be quite aggressive, and will bite or 'pinch' if in contact with skin. They eat other insects, and do, in fact, have chewing mouthparts.

Although Asian lady beetles do not transmit diseases, infestations can trigger allergies in some individuals, ranging from eye irritation to asthma. Because of this, avoid touching your eyes after handling the beetles, and should consult a physician if you think you are having an allergic reaction. Asian lady beetles are also becoming a concern of the wine industry. Due to their noxious odor, even small numbers of beetles inadvertently processed along with grapes can taint the flavor of wine.

The beetles do have a defensive action when threatened or disturbed. They react by forcing some of their tissue fluid through their joints in a behavior called "reflex bleeding." The yellow orange body fluid has a foul odor and can stain clothing and porous surfaces, including walls.

52 ST. JOHN'S WORT – DOES IT WORK?

St. John's Wort is a familiar name to many. There are several species of St. John's Wort (Hypericum species)in Missouri, including Common St. John's Wort, Latin name *hypericum perforatum*. The plant looks like a shrub, and is often found along roadsides in Missouri. It blooms from June – December with yellow blooms comprised of five petals. In fact, St. John's Wort gets its name due to the fact that it begins to flower around the time of the summer solstice on or around June 24, or St. John's day.

In many parts of the world, especially Australia, St. John's Wort is considered a toxic weed. There are reports of it taking over pastures and poisoning livestock. In Australia, a type of beetle has been released to control St. John's Wort in that country, so apparently we aren't the only country that releases beetles or other insects to control noxious plants or insects. Effects on livestock who ingest too much of the plant are due to liver injury and photosensitivity reactions.

St. John's Wort contains the active ingredient, hypericin, which can cause skin reactions when exposed to sunlight, and liver damage in mammals

Medicinal Use

Hypericin also accounts for St. John's Wort use as a natural anti-depressant, an effect which has been studied intensively. The effects are most apparent in mild to moderate depression.

Germany has long been at the forefront of natural cures. My favorite healing salve, Traumeel, orginated in Germany, as did a innovative treatment for autoimminune diseases, called GcMAF. In 1998, a standardized extract from St. John's Wort was developed and improved for treatment of mild and moderate depression. The German Health Authorities recognized early on that the plant was effective in treating depression, but did not approve it until after several years of clinical studies including over 1700 subjects. These studies have shown that the effective dosage is within a range of 600-900 mg extract, with many people having satisfactory effects at the 600 mg per day dosage. Recent pharmacological studies revealed that hypericum extracts work like the selective serotonin reuptake inhibitors (SSRIs), like prozac for example, but to a lesser degree.

Due to the low frequency of side effects when compared with pharmaceutical agents, herbal remedies are growing in popularity among patients, and are more likely to be taken as prescribed. The use of herbal preparations is useful in particular for mild to moderate depression in young patients, and those who want more natural cures. Of all herbal medications, St.-John's Wort has been most widely scientifically documented for the treatment of depression.

St. John's Wort has been around since the first century, and Paracelsus, an early doctor, described it in his writings. Although in modern days St. John's Wort has been used to treat mild to moderate depression, there is exciting new research describing its use as an anti-inflammatory. There are even current investigations using a salve containing St. John's Wort to treat pain and inflammation.

Precautions

Cancer patients who take the herbal remedy St John's Wort may see an impaired response to chemotherapy, particularly the cancer drug irinotecan (Journal of the National Cancer Institute 2002;94:1247-9). St John's Wort has been shown to quickly break down some of the components of cancer medications, ultimately causing a poor response to treatment.

Side effects of St. John's Wort are substantially fewer than synthetic antidepressants, ranging about 3%. The most important risk is photosensitization, which isn't a factor when taken at the recommended dosages.

Marie Lasater

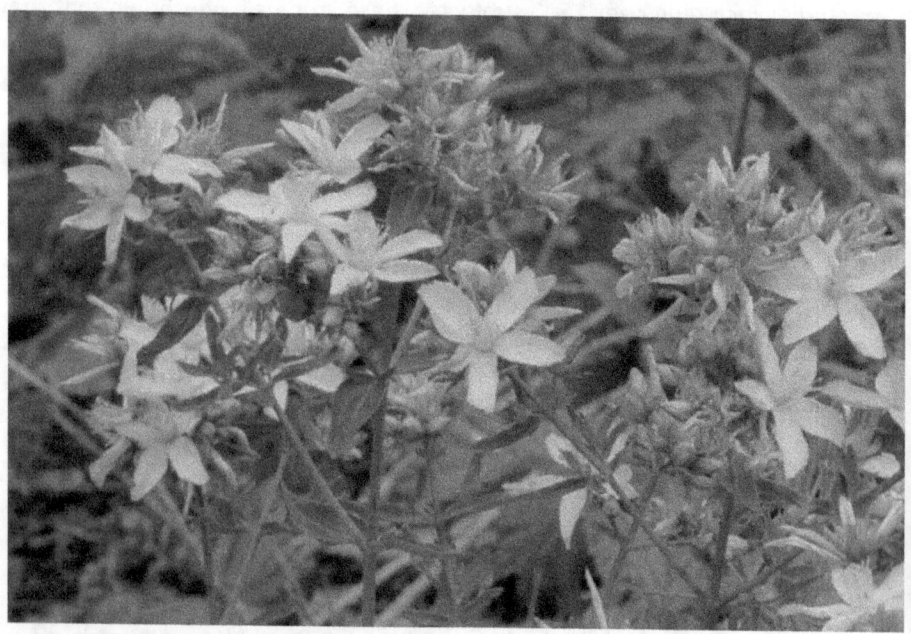

St. John's Wort has bright yellow flowers and grows along roadsides.
Photo by Paul Noll.

53 THE MOST IMPORTANT VITAMIN

Ever wondered why flu season is from October to March? Flu season starts suddenly, peaks, and then ends abruptly. One explanation for this pattern is that the flu may be related to sun exposure, or lack thereof, during the winter months.

Taking it a step further, when we aren't getting any sun, we lose out on Vitamin D; mostly obtained from sun exposure. In fact, our winter levels of Vitamin D can drop to half of our summer levels. Optimal vitamin D levels, seen in people who live in a sun-rich environment year round are between 40-70 ng per ml, but those levels are rarely seen in the current population, so supplements are needed. There are three ways to treat vitamin D deficiency: sunlight, tanning beds, and vitamin D3 supplementation.

Some of the research on Vitamin D and the flu came about by accident. In a study looking at the effect of Vitamin D on preventing osteoporosis, it was found that the subjects in the vitamin D group reported cold and flu symptoms 3 times less often. The third National Health and Nutrition examination survey found a significant decrease in recent upper respiratory tract infections in subjects with adequate Vitamin D levels.

A double blind, placebo-controlled trial comparing vitamin D3 supplements with placebo in schoolchildren to determine if vitamin D supplements during winter and early spring seasons can reduce the incidence of seasonal flu was conducted From December 2008 through March 2009. Children were either given 1200 IU/day of vitamin D vs. placebo (fake pill). The study found a decrease in the incident of Influenza A (10.8%) in the children treated with Vitamin D, vs. 18.6% in children in the placebo group. Further results in children with a previous diagnosis of asthma, asthma attacks occurred in only 2 children receiving vitamin D supplements compared with 12 children receiving placebo.

Vitamin D is more than a vitamin; it is a hormone that boosts our natural immunity. An analysis reviewing 18 randomized controlled trials showed that supplemental Vitamin D, usually in the form of cholecalciferol (vitamin D3) significantly reduces death from many diseases and illnesses. Vitamin D breaks down to a potent hormone, (1.25D) which can trigger a naturally occurring broad-spectrum antibiotic in the body called Cathelicidin that acts as a nature immune defense against invasive bacterial infection.

Dosage and precautions

Treatment of vitamin D deficiency in otherwise healthy patients with 2,000-7,000 IU vitamin D per day should be sufficient to maintain adequate year-round levels of Vitamin D in the body. Higher doses are required in those with serious illnesses associated with vitamin D deficiency, such as cancer, multiple sclerosis, autism, bone degeneration, rheumatoid arthritis, macular degeneration, osteoporosis and periodontal disease, uterine fibroid tumors and even chronic itching. Your local pharmacist can assist you in selecting the correct dosage of this over the counter supplement.

Vitamin D is also produced naturally in the skin after being exposed to ultraviolet B from sunlight (or a tanning bed). When taken as a supplement, the body metabolizes Vitamin D tablets in a similar method to that obtained by the sun. 20,000 IU of Vitamin D can be produced in the skin after just 30 minutes of sun exposure!

The only reason not to take Vitamin D supplements is Vitamin D toxicity or allergy. Obviously, people with skin cancers should avoid sunlight or tanning beds, but oral treatment is fine for these folks.

54 QUICK RELIEF NATURAL CURES

Sometimes you are in a situation where you just need a quick fix for a variety of symptoms. You could be at work, in church, or just in a situation where you only have about 5 minutes to get some relief. Here are six of my top quick fixes that have proven their effectiveness over the years.

Stop Headache Now

This is a technique I learned from my former boss, a board certified neurologist. It works great for migraine headaches, and I've probably recommended it 100 times over the years. First, take a washcloth, wet it, and put some crushed ice in it so it is super cold. Take 2 ibuprofen with 2 aspirin, or 2 tylenol if you prefer, 4 pills total. Sit in a dark room for 5-10 minutes with the cold washrag at the back of your neck, or your forehead. Take the 4 over the counter pills with 1/2 can of Dr. Pepper (no more than 1/2 a can). I've never known this not to work.

Sore Throat

This is an easy one. Put about 1/4 teaspoon of salt in 8 ounces of water, as warm as you can stand it. (Those little salt packets from fast food restaurants work great for this.) Gargle for one minute. The salt water is very healing, but if needed, gargle again as needed.

Blood Pressure

This is a little trickier, but works to get your blood pressure down quickly if you are temporarily out of medication, or waiting to see the doctor. It is NOT a substitute for proper treatment. Using the pads of both thumbs, press on the base of your skull on both sides of your spine. Breathe deeply in and out and count to 30. Next, using your forefingers, draw a line from your head to the top of your skull and press hard while breathing deeply in and out and counting to 30. This will actually hurt where you are applying pressure, and that is to be expected. Last, using you dominant hand, apply as much pressure as you can to the web between your thumb and forefinger on the other hand for another 30 seconds. Wait about 15 minutes and recheck your blood pressure.

Lower back spasms

This is one of my favorites. If you are having lower back pain or spasms, lay on your back with your legs raised and knees bent, Using the second and third fingers of both hands, press the hollow at the back of your knee for about one minute. You should get relief, but if the spasms come back, repeat as necessary.

Toothache

Toothaches can be incapacitating, and are often due to an infection. For many reasons, people can't get to the dentist right away. There is a method that will actually take away the pain, and even treat the infectious process. That method is the century old practice of oil pulling. In order to treat a toothache, use about a tablespoon of sesame oil. Swish the oil in your mouth and around the affected tooth as long as you can, at least 5 minutes, but longer if possible. I say if possible, because there is a chemical change when the oil interacts with your saliva, creating sodium hydroxide. When you spit out the oil, you will notice it has changed to a light creamy brown color and is full of debris from around your possibly infected tooth. Your teeth will also be shiny white; and most of all, the pain will be hugely diminished!

Now you have some tools in your possession when you need quick relief. If you haven't tried these methods before, I'd love to hear your comments on how they work for you.

55 HOME REMEDIES

After just reading about 5 feet of snow overnight in Pennsylvania, and contemplating the not so awful concept of being snowed in for a few days, a review of some tried and true home-based remedies seems to be in order. Here are a few of my go-to tips.

Earache

This works well for children and adults alike, and gives instant, if temporary relief. Hold an ice cube over the affected ear, allowing one drop of melted ice to fall in the ear cavity, where it will reach the tympanic membrane, the sensitive tissue causing the ache.

Alternatively, one drop of a warm essential oil can also be instilled in the ear, but ice seems to work better. Both methods are harmless, and can be repeated.

Flu or cold starting

As soon as possible after feeling symptoms of cold or flu, take 1 tablespoon of apple cider vinegar, once or twice a day. Often this seems to stop the virus in its tracks. Viruses are very stable at acid environments (pH 6.0), but don't like alkaline environments. Although apple cider vinegar is itself acidic, it prompts your body to release hydrogen ions in your urine, raising your pH.

Decongestant

My favorite decongestant has always been, and always will be, pine branch tea. I was feeling a little under the weather just before Christmas, and was about to set out to cut a pine branch to make some tea, when I spotted my Christmas tree. Long story short, tree is missing some branch tips, and I've enjoyed some delicious tea!

Cold Sores

Cold sores are another thing that can be stopped in their tracks with early treatment. If you are prone to cold sores, you a familiar with the little tingle you feel before they break out. Applying tea tree oil to the affected area several times a day will often prevent the virus from replicating, and no sore forms. If the cold sore is already present, applying tea tree oil will lessen healing time by at least 50%, and is much cheaper than other preparations.

Hiccups

Who doesn't hate having the hiccups? For hiccups that just won't quit, nurses have a trick: put a tablespoon of peanut butter on the roof of your mouth. Most of the time, your hiccups will stop in moments.

Nausea

Nausea is a miserable feeling, and that is why I always keep a few cans of Ginger Ale on hand. Eric Yarnell, ND, recommends frozen ginger chips. Chop up fresh ginger, and infuse in hot water. Strain the liquid and freeze in ice cubes trays that make the small cubes to suck on throughout the day. The exact way ginger helps to prevent nausea is unknown, but it has been shown to have an effect on cholinergic receptors that influence nausea, vomiting, and motion sickness.

Chapped Lips

Lips dry, sore and chapped and no chap stick on hand? Use olive oil as an excellent moisturizer.

Snoring

Here's a tip from a neurologist I once worked with. Sew a tennis ball to the back of your pajama top, and if you roll over on your back during sleep, it will wake you up enough to prompt you to roll on your side.

56 AVOIDING ALUMINUM

Aluminum is in flu shots, deodorants, pots and pans, and even rainfall.

Long been suspected in contributing to Alzheimer's disease , aluminum is now implicated in autism. Aluminum is very chemically reactive, and forms solid bonds with fluoride, another neurotoxin. Despite the abundance of aluminum in our environment, no known forms of life use aluminum for any body functions, but it does block absorption of important minerals like iron, magnesium and calcium.

In my own experience, a close friend was having severe pain in his upper arms. It took a little time, but he finally found aluminum-free deodorant, and the arm pain magically went away when he stopped applying aluminum to his armpits. It has been proven that aluminum can easily be absorbed through the skin.

In the average person, the body is able to excrete a small amount of aluminum, but if not excreted, it gets deposited in bone, the brain, abdominal organs, the heart and other muscles where it can cause sickness and even death.

Autism

There have been dozens of published studies in the past year on the relation of aluminum levels in the blood and autism. In November 2017, a study from the University of British Columbia found that there is a link between aluminum additive in vaccines given to children and Autism Spectrum Disorder (ASD). In fact, eight out of 9 Hill Criteria for Causation were documented. To review: Hill's Criteria of Causation documents the minimal conditions needed to establish a causative relation between two items; for example cigarette smoking and lung cancer or emphysema.

Animal studies have demonstrated a range of abnormal behaviors, including abnormalities in social behavior, after postnatal exposure to aluminum. A study published in the Journal of Inorganic Biochemistry concluded, "This is the first experimental study to demonstrate that aluminum can impair social behavior if applied in the early period of postnatal development. The study, however, is insufficient to make any assertive claims about the link between aluminum adjuvants and ASD in humans," as only animals were studied.

Another published study looking at the relationship between aluminum as a vaccine additive found it had a neuro toxic impact on several different neurotransmitters resulting in brain inflammation consistent with autism. Autism is manifested in early childhood, during a window of early developmental vulnerability where the normal developmental trajectory is most susceptible to synthetic chemicals and those not normally found in the human body. The effects are more prevalent in males than females, consistent with some estimates that the male/female ratio in autism is 16:1. Autism spectrum disorders now affect about 1 of every 41 children.

Alzheimer's

Aluminum reduces the rate of growth of human brain cells. In addition to high levels of aluminum found in children with autism, high levels of aluminum have also been found in the brain tissue of Alzheimer patients. An article in the Journal of Alzheimer's Disease states that aluminum is the most abundant neurotoxic metal on earth, repeatedly shown to accumulate in the brains of Alzheimer patients. The report goes on to state the following: 1) very small amounts of aluminum are needed to produce neurotoxicity, 2) aluminum uses different transport mechanisms to cross the blood brain barrier, 3) incremental acquisition of small amounts of Aluminum over a lifetime can result in accumulation in brain tissues, and 4) since 1911, experimental evidence has repeatedly demonstrated that chronic aluminum intake reproduces pathological hallmarks of Alzheimer's, concluding "Immediate steps should be taken to lessen human exposure to aluminum, which may be the single most aggravating and avoidable factor related to Alzheimer's Disease."

Avoiding Aluminum

Get rid of your aluminum pots and pans. Substitute cast iron, glass cookware and stainless steel. The old Revere Ware cookware is invaluable and safe.

Don't use aluminum foil for cooking! Foil is ok to wrap and refrigerate leftovers, but it is even worse than aluminum cookware for cooking. Many aluminum pots are oxidized, with a protective layer (at least when new, and before your scrub the surface off) that prevents aluminum from getting into your food. Aluminum foil has no such protective cover, and allows significant migration of aluminum into food while cooking. Cooking anything acidic accelerates the leaching of aluminum into your food.

Read the label on your deodorant, and purchase only those that are aluminum-free.

57 CELL PHONES, BRAIN TUMORS AND TURMERIC

It is said the best part of cure is prevention. New guidelines released about cell phone use suggest preventative measures to prevent brain tumors.

Have you noticed teens and millennials don't talk on the phone any more? Instead, they text. In my opinion, this is a way our bodies are adapting to the constant attack of radiofrequency waves that are being implicated in the development of brain tumors. Last month, the California Department of Public Health released the following guidelines:

- Keeping the phone away from the body
- Reducing cell phone use when the signal is weak
- Reducing the use of cell phones to stream audio or video, or to download or upload large files
- Keeping the phone away from the bed at night
- Removing headsets when not on a call
- Avoiding products that claim to block radio frequency energy. These products may actually increase your exposure.

California State Public Health Officer Dr. Karen Smith offers, "Children's brains develop through the teenage years and may be more affected by cell phone use. Parents should consider reducing the time their children use cell phones and encourage them to turn the devices off at night."

The International Agency for Cancer Research has classified radiofrequency (RF) radiation, including cell phone radiation, as a possible cancer-causing factor. The brain is especially affected by RF. Data show that if a child starts to use a cell phone at an early age, the probability of brain tumor development at age 29 rises. They recommended children and adolescents younger than sixteen years of age and pregnant women avoid cell phones. It is important to note that RF exposure from a cell phone is higher in the rural areas like ours because of higher output power level needed to communicate with the base station.

There exists extensive evidence that the amount of exposure to cell phone radiation plays a key role in determining the significant associations between cell phone use and gliomas, acoustic neuroma, and meningiomas. Those who use cell phones for more than ten years, more than 20 minutes per day, or cumulative call time for more than 700 hours, have higher risks to develop brain tumors, while those who use cell phones for less than one year have lower risks. Tumors are more likely to be found on the side of the brain where the cell phone is mostly used. Research may explain this effect. In one study, *even with the cell phone turned off,* the region of the brain closest to the phone showed increased brain glucose metabolism. Of course, cancer thrives on glucose (sugar.)

Prevention

What can you do to prevent a possible brain tumor due to constant RF radiation we are constantly exposed to? In addition to following the above-posted guidelines, turmeric has been found in several studies to prevent, and even treat brain tumors. Turmeric is not very soluble, so large doses are typically needed to have a therapeutic effect, In animals given injections of turmeric, it has been found to block brain tumor formation and also eliminates brain tumor cells.

Curcumin is found in turmeric root, a member of the ginger family. It is used for several disorders, and recently there has been a lot of research regarding its role in treating brain tumors. It attack brain cancer in several ways, including inducing death of cancer cells, decreasing spread of cancer cells, increasing the efficiency of chemotherapy, interrupting mitochondria in the cancer cell and blocking signals that help to keep cancer cells alive. It may affect the stem cells in tumors associated with a high grade and poor prognosis.

As noted above, the problem with turmeric is poor absorption into the body. Case reports of brain cancer patients who have had success with turmeric took large doses several times per day. Turmeric has a low toxicity, even at high doses. There are currently over 100 clinical trials throughout the world recruiting subjects to assess the beneficial effects of turmeric.

58 WHY YOU SHOULD SAVE YOUR BABY'S TEETH

Recently on Facebook there was a post about a baby tooth monster doll. In fact these dolls aren't made with human teeth at all, but individual false teeth. They are creepy though.

Every mother I know feels compelled to save their children's baby teeth. This is a very good practice, as a child's baby tooth stores a lot of valuable and irreplaceable information. For example, in March of 2013 the Greater St. Louis Citizens' Committee for Nuclear Information (CNI) presented the first scientific report of the Baby Tooth Survey that was conducted in the St. Louis area from 1958 - 1970. The released study showed how much strontium-90 was absorbed from 1951 – 1954.

Following nuclear testing in the mid-1950's, an untold number of both military and unsuspecting civilians died after exposure to nuclear radiation. Women, especially mothers, took the lead in investigating the impact of nuclear testing. Beginning in 1958, St. Louis' Nuclear Women organized the CNI, mentioned above.

As one of the first "citizen-scientist collaborations," dentistry professors from Washington University School of Dentistry began the scientific study of baby teeth of children submitted by mothers and children alike, finding that "radioactive strontium-90 levels in the baby teeth of children born from 1945 to 1965 had risen 100-fold and that the level of strontium-90 rose and fell in correlation with atomic bomb tests.

During that period, there was significant rise in childhood cancers, prompting President Kennedy to negotiate a treaty with Russia to end above-ground testing of atomic bombs on August 5th, 1963, a mere three months before he was assassinated. Despite the treaty, data from ongoing tests on baby teeth showed that recent underground nuclear detonations were venting radiation into the water, soil and sky. The whole time, the Atomic Energy Commission denied nuclear fallout had any effect on humans. By the end of Baby Tooth Survey in 1970, almost 300,000 teeth had been collected and analyzed; and baby teeth don't lie.

How did Strontium-90 get into the teeth? One theory is that there is a "milk pathway" by which fallout from nuclear testing in the 1950s and 1960s contaminated pastures, and the milk of cows that grazed there. Strontium, like fluoride, replaces calcium in bone and teeth. Other minerals that replace calcium include cadmium and phosphorus.

According to a recent study, baby teeth contain an abundance of stem cells, a very special type of cell that can potentially grow replacement tissue in the body and cure a number of diseases.

The original baby tooth study ended in 1970, and went dormant for several years before coming back on track in 2009, when research queries were sent to thousands of tooth donors from over 50 years ago, seeking health data on the long-term effects of Strontium. The half-life of radioactive strontium-90 is 28.79 years, close to that of cesium-137; making it detectable in human teeth for several decades.

Recent research has found a way to extract stem cells from some saved baby teeth, especially those that fall out on their own; stem cells that may be crucial to treat a rare disease if cord blood wasn't saved following birth.

In a case in Australia, DNA extracted from a baby tooth helped solve the unknown cause of death of a little girl. Following years of grief and worry, DNA established the cause of death as Rett Syndrome, a rare, unpreventable neurologic disorder, giving the child's parents some answers.

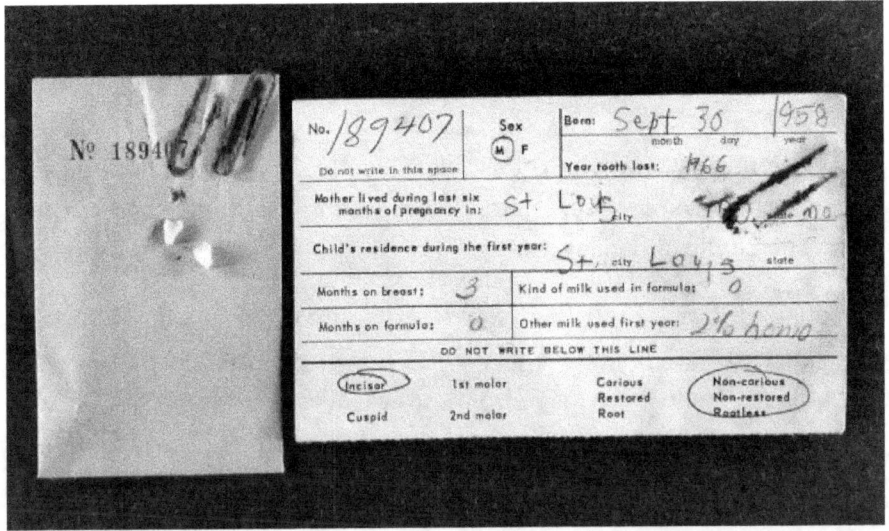

Picture of a tooth, the info card, and the original envelope that were part of the strontium studies in baby teeth that have been stored for years at Washington University's Tyson Research Center in southwest St. Louis County. (Retrieved from Internet: http://www.stltoday.com/news/local/baby-tooth-survey-radiation-fallout-checkup-is-on/article_75514385-d829-5bda-8ee1-098363dfeab6.html

59 COFFEE LEAF TEA

As a youngster, I wrote to the Folger's coffee company, and they sent me a small coffee tree. It grew quite well in the house, and had the most beautiful green leaves.

Coffee is loved throughout the world, with people naturally dividing themselves into tea drinkers or coffee drinkers. Fortunately, you can be both! Yes, there is tea made from coffee leaves; it turns out they are not just pretty foliage. Coffee leaves are a rich source of mangiferin, also found in mango leaves, which are a little bit harder to come by.

Mangiferin has many health benefits, including managing diabetes, anti-cancer agent, anti-viral, memory enhancer, protection against radiation, to name a few.

Antidiabetic

Mangiferin lowers blood sugar and has other antidiabetic properties. In one study, diabetes was induced in animals via a high-fat/high fructose diet for eight weeks who were then treated with mangiferin for 28 days. The effects of mangiferin were compared to the pharmaceutic medication for diabetes, Avandia, and found to have similar positive effects on obesity, elevated blood sugar and insulin resistance. The researchers concluded that "the results obtained in this study provide evidence that mangiferin is a possible beneficial natural compound for type 2 diabetes and metabolic disorders associated with the metabolic syndrome."

Gastric cancer

A study published in December 2017 investigated the effects of mangiferin on gastric carcinoma cells, and the way in which they were affected. They found that mangiferin slowed proliferation and caused cell death in gastric cancer cells, in both a time and dose dependent manner.

Antiviral

Mangiferin has remarkable anti-viral action against HSV-I (herpes virus). It was overwhelmingly found that mangiferin is superior to such control drugs as acyclovir, a common herpes drug. The antiviral effect of mangiferin was attributed presumably its ability to inhibit virus replication within cells.

Memory

Studies on multiple types of memory loss, including that associated with Alzheimers, long-term memory and recognition, show that mangiferin improves memory through a mechanism that might involve an increase in neurotrophin and cytokine levels in the brain.

Radiation protection

Mangiferin protects against several types of radiation, including X-ray, gamma, and ultraviolet. It is frequently added to cosmetics, due to its antioxidant and ultraviolet protection.

Obesity

Not only do the leaves of the coffee plant contain Mangiferin, they also contain caffeine. Recent science is showing that caffeine is not so bad after all, as long is it is consumed in moderation.

When treating obesity, not much has been understood about the effect of caffeine. Recent studies show that caffeine can contribute to weight loss through a couple of ways: by blocking the development of new fat cells through thermogenesis (creation of heat) that reduces the size and number of fat cell so fat doesn't accumulate.

Coffee Beans

Let's not forget coffee beans. Especially delicious when covered in healthy dark chocolate, compounds found in coffee beans can protect against respiratory viruses.

As noted above, coffee leaves have antiviral activity against herpes simplex viruses. Green coffee beans have also been found to have mild effects against both the adenovirus and influenza virus. In a recent study when coffee beans were evaluated against RSV (respiratory syncytial virus), there was a potent antiviral effect, "warranting clinical development as a potential anti-respiratory syncytial virus drug" from coffee beans.

Precautions:

Mangiferin acts as an efficient iron chelator, removing iron from the body, so those with iron deficiency anemia should use caution.

60 IMPROVING YOUR VISION WITHOUT GLASSES - PART 1

More and more young people need glasses; and for everyone, it seems each trip to the eye doctor requires a progressively stronger prescription. At least partly to blame for our universal vision loss is the amount of time we spend staring at a television set, a computer screen, or a cell phone. Merely interacting with electronic devices deprives us of the basic experience of vision, as our eyes turn into mere transmitters of digital information.

Think about the last time you paused to soak in a beautiful sight. Now, think about how often your eyes are used merely to read, write, check facebook, watch TV, etc. When was the last time your eyes saw exactly what your mind was seeing, but instead presented you problems to work on? As an example, go outside right now and look around for 15 seconds. Come back inside, and describe what your mind recorded. Next, try it again, RELAX, and spend a few minutes really seeing your surroundings. For Navy men, living for months in a submarine where their distance vision can be limited to looking only about 15 feet, it has been found that their eyes adapt for close vision, with the shape of the eyeball literally changing shape, limiting their range of sight.

A new problem that has arisen is temporary one-sided vision loss. Generally, sudden vision loss in one eye is an emergency condition. The new condition was reported in 2016 in the New England Journal of Medicine when two women went temporarily blind after checking their backlit electronic devices while lying in bed in the dark. Both women experienced recurring temporary vision loss in one eye, lasting up to 15 minutes, while lying on their side n the dark, looking at their phone or tablet with only one eye open. When neurological examinations, including MRI, were normal, physician Dr. Plant explained it by saying "So you have one eye adapted to the light because it's looking at the phone and the other eye is adapted to the dark," he said. When they put their phone down, they couldn't see with the phone eye, because "it's taking many minutes to catch up to the other eye that's adapted to the dark." This temporary blindness can be avoided by keeping both eyes open when looking at the device, but that is generally uncomfortable due to the brightness of the backlight, and certainly not good for your vision.

In 1919, Doctor William Bates, a renowned physician who dedicated his life to studying vision, published a revolutionary book called "The Bates Method for Better Eyesight Without Glasses," which is still popular today. Doctor Bates concluded that the driving forces for good vision are the eye muscles that can lengthen or shorten the whole eyeball, not just the lens. This theory is supported by the fact that people can see clearly even if the lens in the eye is not present, as with cataract surgery. Dr. Bates has some other radical theories for his time, including the claim that vision can be healed through rehabilitation, much like a broken bone, and that glasses are similar to crutches, only needed until healing occurs.

The Bates program includes a comprehensive collection of home treatments to improve vision. Next week, we will review some of these exercises, and how they can benefit your eyesight.

61 IMPROVING YOUR VISION WITHOUT GLASSES - PART 2

It is as natural for the eye to see as it is for the mind to acquire knowledge, and any effort in either case is not only useless, but defeats the end in view.

~Wm H Bates: Perfect Sight Without Glasses, published 1920

Vision loss is usually considered irreversible because the retina and optic nerve do not repair themselves like some of the other parts of the body. There is hope, however, because of the huge role the brain plays in vision. For those with low vision, the brain takes in and interprets visual information, and has the ability to enhance vision where it is interpreted by the brain through an amazing ability we all possess, called neuroplasticity. Think of how much we have learned over the years. Without the ability of the brain to grow and change, our mind would change little from that of a newborn infant. For us older folks, the brain actually grows stronger with age, if we keep it stimulated and challenged. Throughout our entire life, our brain remains plastic (changeable).

Research is being conducted on how plasticity can be used to activate residual vision for the treatment of visual field loss in conditions like glaucoma, diabetic retinopathy or optic neuropathy. Almost all people have some residual vision, and the goal of therapy is to strengthen existing vision; including enlarging the visual field, improving reaction time, and improving vision related quality of life that includes acuity, reading, mobility or orientation. About 70 % of the patients respond to the therapies and there are no serious adverse events.

New treatment programs have been tested in clinical studies, including vision restoration training and non-invasive alternating current stimulation. Both methods have been shown to improve vision. Treatment with alternating current stimulation (30 min. daily for 10 days) activates and stimulates the entire retina and brain. The procedure involves attaching four electrodes around patients' eyes. A current is then emitted that travels directly to the brain. In a 2016 study using this method, eyesight improved by an average of 24%, and patients reported being able to read small print again.

Unlike alternating current stimulation, vision restoration training can be performed at home, once you know the exercises.

Below are discussed what I consider the two most popular vision restoration techniques, and are part of the Bates Vision Program.

Blinking: Palm your hands over your closed eyes, completely blocking out light. and set to allow the eyes to blink freely. Blink for 3- - 60 seconds, then relax and repeat. Frequent blinking is always good throughout the day, and is necessary to clean and moisten the eyes.

Directional Eye Movements: There are several ways to accomplish exercising your eye muscles. Fixing your vision a few yards away, imagine a large clock, the type you had in grade school. Using only your eyes, look at each number 1 -12 on the clock. Taking your eyes through a full range of motion. Next, focus on a pencil, and while facing straight ahead, move the pencil left and right to the edge of your vision, following it using only your eyes. Do the same thing going up and down, and from the upper left corner to the lower right corner of your vision and reversing from the upper right corner to the lower left corner. You will instantly feel more alert. This is a great one-minute break to take when working at a computer screen all day.

62 CHEMTRAILS

By Tamara Glascock

There is much discussion these days about chemtrails. Are they the same thing as contrails? Are they harmful to our health or environment? Can we protect ourselves from them?

According to the dictionary, there isn't a whole lot of difference between chemtrails and contrails. So, how does one distinguish the difference? Contrails, which are said to be nothing more than water condensation, are seen as a short white trail left behind as an aircraft flies overhead. It dissipates quickly, and is said to be completely harmless to both humans and the environment.

Chemtrails are seen as long white trails left behind an aircraft, that linger for extended periods of time, often hours, gradually changing from a thin white line, (or a criss-cross checkerboard pattern), growing thicker and fluffier as they spread out, eventually resembling puffy white clouds before thinning out and disappearing. They contain several toxic chemicals that are known to damage both humans and the environment.

Recent studies of air, water and soil quality from across the United States have shown alarmingly elevated levels of toxic chemicals and heavy metals that are believed to be a result of chemtrails, among other things. Aluminum, strontium 90, barium and "chaff" (mylar fibers like those found in fiberglass, coated with aluminum, desiccated blood cells, plastic, and paper), are believed to be a few of the toxins contained in chemtrails. It is believed by many that chemtrails are causing mutations in plant life, and polluting our water supply.

Aluminum has an affinity for water and easily binds to all life forms. It can be absorbed into water, earth, plants, and humans. It can attach to moisture in the air that we then breath in. Aluminum is a known contributor to diseases such as Alzheimer's and other neurological disorders, cancer, respiratory diseases, gastrointestinal issues, and immune system failure. Combined with other heavy metals like cadmium and barium, both of which are believed to be present in chemtrails, you have a dangerous cocktail of toxic chemicals that you are ingesting daily.

With all these problems, and to quote Dane Wigington at geoengineeringwatch.org, why on earth are they spraying? Many think it is to mitigate the effects of global warming. On clear days following heavy spraying, you can often see a ray of blazing hot sunlight peeking through. Another theory is weather manipulation, the creating of rain and snow. Keep in mind that weather is a commodity on the futures market. Weather moderation has been around a long time. Remember the 1956 film, The Rainmaker? In late 1915, San Diego hired a "moisture accelerator" named Charles Hatfield during a drought. He seeded the clouds with his own chemical concoction, and on January 1, 1916, it started raining in San Diego and didn't stop until February. The 30 inches of rain that fell destroyed the dams and railroad tracks, caused massive property damage, and killed up to 50 citizens. Weather modification has been around a long time.

While there is little that can be done to prevent this from happening, it is possible to protect ourselves from the devastating effects of chemtrails. Our first line of defense is a strong immune system. Eating foods as clean as possible is key. Organic, fresh fruits and vegetables provide a majority of the vitamins and nutrients the body needs to stay healthy. To help counter the effects of heavy metals such as aluminum, eat dark greens (like spinach and kale), green peppers, asparagus, beets, and sunflower seeds that contain high levels of silicon dioxide. However, even organic produce is taking a hit from the fallout of the chemtrails, so be sure to thoroughly wash them in warm water with a drop or two of natural soap, or rinse them in a mixture of ¼ cup vinegar and 1 cup of water to remove any toxic residue.

A good heavy metal cleanse will help remove many of the toxic chemicals and metals from your body. I suggest a good cleanse 2-3 times per year, even if you aren't experiencing any ill effects. When choosing a cleanse, look for something that contains naturally-detoxifying ingredients like burdock root, dandelion root, activated charcoal, milk thistle, red clover, stinging nettle, cilantro, parsley, and psyllium seed. These ingredients will help draw toxins from your organs and bloodstream so the body can more easily dispose of them through the elimination system. They will also help stimulate the organs to work properly without causing undue stress, and are all extremely safe when used properly.

If you still don't believe chemtrails are real, check out the hundreds of patents for geo-engineering at the U.S. Patent office.

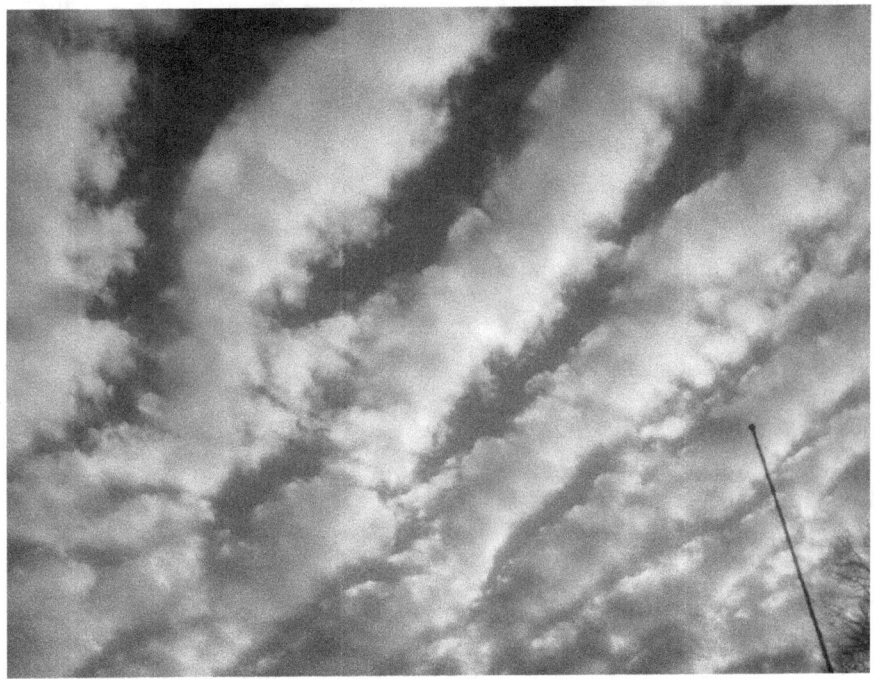

Chemtrails south of Rolla.

63 PINE POLLEN

In a few months, it will be all around us. If you have pine trees on your place, you are familiar with waking up to your vehicle covered with a fine yellow powder. That is pine pollen. Believe it or not, many people go to great lengths to harvest pollen directly from the tree, using a variety of methods that include standing under a pollen laden tree and shaking the pollen into a large bag. Before its release, the pollen is held in catkins on the tree. Catkins look like a yellow pine cone, and get their name from the Dutch katteken (kitten), as some think they resemble a kitten's tail.

Why on earth would anybody harvest pine pollen? It is actually a super food, containing 18 amino acids (the building blocks of protein), and is full of minerals and vitamins A, B complex, C, E, and Beta-carotene. It also provides Vitamin. D, rare for plants! After harvesting, fresh pollen is stable for as long as 24 hours. Prior to storage, moisture content must be reduced to less than 10%. It can then be held in a refrigerator at 37° F (refrigerator temperature) for up to 1 year in a container that maintains low moisture content.

Medicinal uses

In addition to over 200 nutrients readily absorbed from the body, pine pollen contains beneficial enzymes and powerful antioxidants and natural plant-based steroids. Pine pollen also reduces lipofuscin deposits which affect the heart, brain and liver.

Antioxidant

Antioxidants are good because they slow down the aging process, and get rid of free radicals, toxic byproducts produced in response to some of the conditions we experience in our day to day life, include ultraviolet exposure. Pine pollen does this by increasing levels of superoxide dismutase, a master antioxidant, and increasing glutathione that helps to detoxify pollutants in the environment.

Testosterone for androgen/estrogen balance

Pine Pollen also contains bioavailable forms of androgen, testosterone and DHEA which, unlike synthetic steroids, have less side effects because they are natural. Androgens are to men what estrogen is to women, making pine pollen supplements a favorite of body builders as it promotes the growth of lean muscle. Androgens from pine pollen are nearly identical to those found in the human body.

Even for women, testosterone can be helpful to middle aged adults whose bodies are making less of the hormone. With older women, testosterone can improve mood and feelings of well-being.

Lipofuscin deposits.

As mentioned above, pine pollen reduces lipofuscin deposits which affect the heart, brain and liver. Wikipedia describes lipofuscin quite nicely as "the name given to fine yellow-brown pigment granules composed of lipid-containing residues of lysosomal digestion. It is considered to be one of the aging or "wear-and-tear" pigments, found in the liver, kidney, heart muscle, retina, adrenals, nerve cells, and ganglion cells." Obviously not something you want lingering in your organs.

Recipes

There are dozens of ways to use pine pollen. Stir 1/4 teaspoon into your oatmeal, or add to a soup or smoothie. If you make your own pasta, pine pollen can be substituted for part of the flour.

Allergies

What about allergies? Pine pollen allergies are less common than other allergies, but the sap can cause allergies upon contact with skin. Pine nuts can result in serious allergic reactions, but those are generally found on commercially grown pines.

64 JERUSALEM ARTICHOKE: DIABETICS TAKE NOTE

In a previous column, we discussed the role of the Jerusalem Artichoke, *Helianthus tuberosus*, as a food source. Native to Missouri, the plant blooms from July through October, and is readily visible along the roadside, growing up to 10 feet with multiple flower heads per stem; not to mention a distinguishing chocolate scent.

Popular since the 1600's, in the last 10 years a new emphasis has been placed on the medicinal properties of Jerusalem Artichoke in regards to its anti-diabetic properties; in addition, it is a great source of fiber and sugar substitute for people who require insulin. There is growing demand for different products, including food, biofuels, medicine, animal nutrition, and processing of inulin derived from the plant.

Inulin

Inulin is a starchy substance found in some plants, with Jerusalem Artichoke and chicory being the most common. According to Web MD, the inulin that is used for medicine is most commonly obtained by soaking chicory roots in hot water.

The medicinal uses of inulin include reducing blood cholesterol and triglycerides, and like insulin, inulin helps to lower blood glucose and reduce weight. In the food industry, it is used as a natural additive to improve the taste of some manufactured foods. Inulin is considered a functional food ingredient as it affects both the physiological and biochemical processes in the body, resulting in better health and reduction in the risk of many diseases, and does this in several ways.

Immune protection

Not absorbed until it gets to the bowel, inulin acts as a probiotic, where beneficial bacteria utilize it, and it decreases disease-causing bacteria, just one of the ways inulin stimulates the immune system. Diets including inulan have been associated with a reduced chance of colon cancer. It also relieves constipation naturally.

Blood sugar regulation

In one study conducted with horses, inulin was added to horse feed, including oat grains and meadow hay. After 3 weeks of this diet, both glucose and insulin levels declined more rapidly until four hours after the feeding, and tended to stay lower.

Obesity

Of course, to lose weight, reducing your calorie intake is essential. One way to do this is by increasing your fiber intake, and a high fiber diet helps you to feel full.

The fructose found in Jerusalem artichoke belongs to the dietary fiber category. One study looked at the effects of a 2,000 calorie per day diet that included Jerusalem artichoke concentrate in obese teens and adults. 12 obese students (6 boys and 6 girls) and 6 obese women were put on a low-calorie regimen for 12 weeks, while 16 obese students (10 boys and 6 girls) and 17 obese women consumed the same low-calorie diet that included Jerusalem artichoke concentrate. The subjects self-reported their feeling of fullness after eating. In addition to measuring weight and body fat percentage, serum biomarkers of lipid and carbohydrate metabolism and adipokines (substances secreted by fat tissue that cause obesity related diseases) were determined.

The 2000 calorie a day diet completed with Jerusalem artichoke concentrate resulted in a diminished sensation of hunger. Body mass index and body fat percentage decreased significantly. In girls and women, the serum levels of triglycerides were also significantly reduced and the rate of insulin resistance was decreased. The researchers concluded, "results of this pilot study appear to demonstrate that the Jerusalem artichoke concentrate produced by a new technology can be a promising component of future diet therapy."

Other health benefits

Inulin found in Jerusalem Artichoke reduces the risk of osteoporosis by increasing mineral absorption, especially calcium, and reduces the risk of hardening of the arteries by lowering the production of triglycerides and fatty acids in the liver and decreasing their level in the blood.

65 MISSOURI WINTERGREEN

Remember Teaberry gum when you were a kid? It got its name from the common name of the wintergreen plant that grows throughout the eastern United States. Although Wintergreen wasn't used to make the gum, the flavor resembled that of the plant.

Wintergreen (*Gaultheria procumbens*), is a great garden plant, used as a ground cover in part shade to full shade, and does best in USDA hardiness zones 3 to 8; Missouri is zone 4 to 7. It grows naturally in wooded areas and clearings. The plant flowers from June – July, with bell shaped white flowers that produce bright red berries that last all winter. Both the leaves and fruit smell and taste like the round pink candies you may remember as a kid.

Leaves from the wintergreen plant have been used since antiquity to make oil of wintergreen. A popular science experiment uses oil of wintergreen as a base ingredient with which to manufacture aspirin (acetylsalicylic acid) due to its high content of methyl salicylate that metabolizes to salicylic acid.

Wintergreen has been a popular flavoring for chewing gum, candy and chewing tobacco. Native Americans used the dried leaves to make tea, hence the common name "Teaberry." Due to its natural aspirin content, poultices and salves containing oil of wintergreen are great for applying directly to the skin for sore muscles and arthritis. The fruit of the plant can be safely eaten, but concentrated oil of wintergreen has been shown to cause death if consumed, more about that later.

Oil of Wintergreen has astringent and antiseptic properties, which in addition to the pleasant taste, make it a popular ingredient in toothpaste and mouthwashes. It is used in small amounts as an antiseptic in Listerine, and is thought to kill the bacteria *streptococcus mutans,* which are implicated in causing cavities.

Other Uses

Wintergreen oil also has a place in fine art, where it is used to transfer a color laser print to a canvas. The printed image is coated with wintergreen oil, then transferred onto canvas by pressing it face down under pressure using an etching press. Other applications include use as a non-toxic lubricant in firearm maintenance.

Toxicity

Oil of Wintergreen can be very toxic if ingested in sufficient quantity. In 1985, an 81-year-old man died at Vanderbilt Hospital when he was accidentally given a fatal dose of oil of wintergreen used by the housekeeping for cleaning. The oil of wintergreen was stored in a bottle kept in the refrigerator with the medication he was prescribed. Poison Control warns that 1 teaspoon of concentrated *wintergreen oil* (98%) equals 7 grams of aspirin, about 21 tablets, which can cause death due to salicylate poisoning. The symptoms include sweating, nausea, vomiting, ringing in the ears and hyperventilation. This is a cautionary tale; just because a medicine comes from a plant, it can still be toxic, as is the case with bloodroot, sold locally as Tumor-Be-Gone, and for which a man is currently sitting in prison.

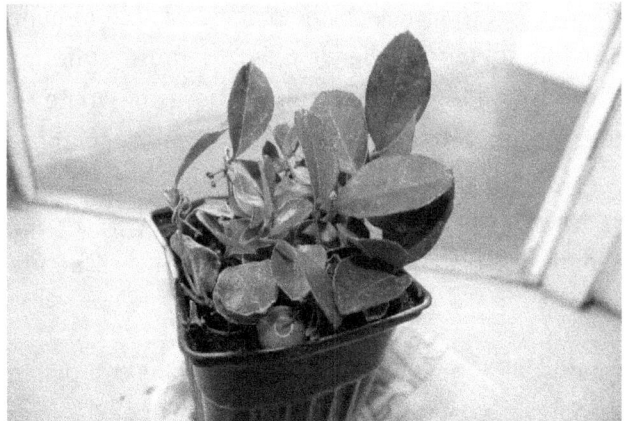

Native Wintergreen has dark green leaves with a glossy finish and cherry-like berries.

66 THE MANY USES OF RAW HONEY

By: Tamara Glascock

Raw honey. Everyone has heard of all the benefits, so much so that we may tend to tune out when the subject is brought up. Yes, it truly is that wonderful. It really does boost the immune system, heal wounds, treat burns, boosts energy, calms allergies, and basically makes us nearly immortal.

Knowing all that doesn't really mean much if we don't know how to use it properly to treat each of those conditions, though. Let's cover a few basics first, just in case you haven't learned all of this before.

Raw honey means that it is unfiltered and unheated. This is important when it comes to gaining the health benefits. Honey is made by bees from the pollen of all the plants growing near their home. Those little nuggets of pollen are absorbed into the honey. If your honey is heated, it destroys not only those beneficial bits of pollen, but all of the other healing properties contained in the honey. When it is filtered, that means that all of those little nuggets are separated from the honey. Those nuggets of pollen are responsible for helping boost the immune system, and they are the source of allergy relief to those suffering seasonal allergies by exposing the person to minute doses of whatever pollen is causing the issue, thereby building up an immunity to those allergens. Typically, 1 Tablespoon per day is suggested, but I advise taking 1 Tablespoon twice a day. It generally takes 6-8 weeks to see relief from allergy symptom, so be patient! Start taking it well before allergy season hits.

This is also why buying local honey is important. You want the pollen that you are exposed to every day to be from the same source that is causing the problem. Local does not mean the honey has to be from your neighborhood. Your county would be perfectly fine. Your state would be acceptable. Your geographical region works in a pinch. As long as it is raw and local, you will be gaining the greatest benefit..

Honey is made up of 80% natural sugars, 18% water, and a whole passel of vitamins, minerals and proteins. If you are looking for a jump-start in the morning, or for a quick energy boost throughout the day, try adding a teaspoon or two to your water, fresh juice or smoothie. Honey has been referred to as the perfect running fuel for athletes because it supplies a form of energy that is easily absorbed by the body, along with carbohydrates that are needed pre-and post-exercise. So, you can ditch the costly energy and protein drinks and take a shot of honey instead!

Feeling a bit under the weather? Before running to the doctor or ER the next time you feel an illness coming on, boost your immune system naturally. Honey's antibiotic, antibacterial, anti-fungal and anti-inflammatory properties are undisputed. Mix equal parts raw honey and either raw apple cider vinegar or fresh lemon juice. Throw in 1" section of raw, grated ginger, 4-5 cloves of pressed, fresh garlic and add a tiny pinch of cayenne. It has been our experience that this works faster than a round of antibiotics, and provides many additional benefits without a single negative side effect. The addition of the vinegar, ginger, garlic and cayenne provide a balanced, powerful boost, not only the immune system, but to the entire body.

The same qualities that make it the perfect substitute for antibiotics make it ideal for burn and wound care, too. Hospitals around the world have used honey as a dressing for wounds and burns with phenomenal results. It is as simple as smearing raw honey on the damaged area and covering it with a bandage that gets changed every 24-48 hours. The honey reacts with the body fluids to create a natural form of hydrogen peroxide that kills harmful bacteria, and delivers the same antibacterial and antibiotic properties directly to the damaged area. Whether you have a small rash or a deep wound or burn, honey helps soothe pain, and helps heal the damage, and helps the body create new cells to replace the damaged ones.

67 THE MANY USES OF RAW HONEY – PART 2

By Tamara Glascock – guest writer

Is your hair looking dull and lifeless? Add a few tablespoons to ½ cup of coconut oil, rub it into your hair and scalp. Let it sit for 30 minutes to an hour, then rinse it out with warm water or a mild, natural shampoo. Honey is a natural humectant that will help restore moisture and shine to hair. The coconut oil, with all of its amazing health benefits, will help repair damaged, dry hair, helps balance the pH of the scalp, clears up dandruff, and helps carry the honey deeper into the skin and hair.

You know that persistent, nasty cough that just won't go away, despite having tried every cough syrup on the market and a round or two of antibiotics? Try honey. Increasing scientific evidence shows that a single dose of honey can reduce mucus secretion and coughs. In one study, honey was just as effective as diphenhydramine (benadryl) and dextromethorphan, common ingredients found in over-the counter cough medicines. Want to add a bit of oomph to your honey? Infuse it with cloves of fresh garlic, some yarrow blossoms, a bit of marshmallow root, ginger root, or some wild cherry bark. Let it sit in a cool, dark place for 6-8 weeks, stirring it occasionally.

Insomnia hits us all from time to time. A dose of honey before bed can be helpful in two ways. Honey restocks the liver's glycogen supply; preventing the brain from thinking it needs fuel, which can cause you to wake up prematurely. Even more helpful, though, is that honey prompts the brain to release melatonin. This happens by creating spikes in insulin levels, which stimulates the release of tryptophan, which is converted to serotonin, then melatonin. The process is a bit complicated, but the results are not. As a bonus, melatonin does more than promote restful sleep. It also boosts the immune system and helps the body rebuild damaged tissue during periods of sleep. With better sleep comes more health benefits in the form of less stress, less anxiety, lower blood pressure and cholesterol levels, heart health, and much more. So, no need for any more OTC sleep aids that can cause more serious health issues, and can cause you to wake up feeling less-than-rested, groggy or irritable.

Some of the most interesting research on honey has come from the cancer arena. Honey contains a disease-fighting antioxidant flavonoid called pinocembrin, Pinocembrin supports enzyme activity, and many studies have shown that pinocembrin induces apoptosis (programmed cell death) of many types of cancer cells. Further, honey is capable of acting like a trojan horse, making it especially useful when treating brain issues like dementia, brain cancer and tumors, and brain trauma. The body sees the honey as a source of glucose and allows it to penetrate both cells and the blood-brain barrier. When the honey is infused with other ingredients, like herbs that are known to kill cancer cells, it is able to deliver the healing properties directly to the damaged cells without harming healthy ones. In the case of brain issues, this is especially beneficial because the brain is endowed with so many barriers that were designed to protect it that medical science has had a difficult time finding safe ways to work around it without doing more harm than good.

Raw honey has so much to offer us in the way of health benefits. Regardless of what your health issues may be, 1-2 Tablespoons of honey per day may be the answer you have been searching for!

68 THE NATURAL PAIN MEDICATION YOU'VE NEVER HEARD OF

By: Tamara Glascock

Mitragyna speciosa, commonly known as kratom, and a close relative of the coffee plant, has a controversial past and an uncertain future. The leaf of the plant is commonly used to treat chronic pain and anxiety, but its most notable application is in helping opioid drug users to withdraw from illicit drugs. In 2016, a small bipartisan group of House lawmakers asked the Drug Enforcement Administration to place the herbal supplement mitragyna onto Schedule I of the Controlled Substances Act, a label that would place it in the same category as LSD, heroin, and marijuana. The reasons cited were "a high potential for abuse and no current medical use." Public outcry, combined with the overwhelming evidence of its usefulness as a valuable, safe medicine kept that from happening. Yet, mitragyna has been proactively banned by two states, and the active ingredient, mitragynine, has been banned in four states as opponents continue the push to have it labeled as a dangerous drug.

Amid all of this controversy, one might think that mitragyna was the cause of serious health issues, hospitalizations, or even a few deaths. In truth, mitragyna has never been implicated in any reported adverse long-term health issues when used properly. It has been reported as the cause of death in 44 cases worldwide, but this number is incredibly misleading. According to official FDA reports, in nearly every case the individual had other known deadly substances in their system at the time of death, including synthetic opiates, benzodiazepines, anti-depressants and, in one case, a medication used to treat his Tourette's syndrome. In a bizarre case, the cause of death was a gunshot wound to the chest. Since mitragyna was found in the system the FDA listed it as a contributing factor.

The opioid crisis that has swept the country has brought with it a conservatively-estimated $11 billion per year profit for pharmaceutical companies, which could go far in explaining the controversy surrounding this plant and its promising use as an effective, safe opiate alternative, as well as its record of successfully treating opiate-withdrawal. The newly-appointed head of the FDA, Scott Gottlieb's financial disclosure form shows that he made approximately $3 million throughout 2016 through a combination of speaking fees, consulting arrangements with drug companies, board memberships, and his work at healthcare-focused investment firms. As the guest speaker before such entities as Healthcare Distributors Alliance, a trade group for the largest opioid wholesale distributors in America, and Mallinckrodt Pharmaceuticals, the maker of a highly-addictive generic oxycodone pill, as well as seven other pharmaceutical companies in 2015, combined with a recent interview on CNBC in which he stated that the FDA does not believe kratom to have any value on the opioid front, proponents of mitragyna are concerned that the battle to keep it legal is not over yet.

All of this may leave you wondering what all the fuss is about, and if you should avoid using mitragyna altogether. One of the country's foremost addiction specialists, Johns Hopkins University's Dr. Jack Henningfield, stated "It's important to understand that although mitragyna has some mild effects similar to opioids, its chemical make-up is different, and it appears overall much safer. In fact, mitragyna's analgesic effects and impact on energy, combined with its favorable safety profile supports continued access by consumers to appropriately regulated mitragyna products while research on its uses continues."

Walter C. Prozialeck, PhD, chairman of the department of pharmacology at Midwestern University in Illinois, said, "If it lived up to its billing, some of the compounds in kratom could be useful at least as the basis for the development of better drugs that would treat pain without the addictive benefit of opioids. That would be an amazing advance in pain management," Prozialeck says. "But nobody knows how research will turn out. It could be a dead end. The biggest negative of the DEA ban is it will stifle any research in this area."

Next week we will discuss how mitragyna works, where it grows, and therapeutic effects.

69 THE NATURAL PAIN MEDICATION YOU'VE NEVER HEARD OF – PART 2

By Tamara Glascock

As we discussed last week, it is very likely you've never heard of mitragyna speciosa. The plant grows mainly in Thailand, where it is a huge export product.

The primary active alkaloid in mitragyna leaves, mitragynine, is responsible for its opioid-like effects, and opponents of the herb believe this substance could, possibly, cause dependence. Remember that mitragyna is in the coffee family, and does not bind as strongly to the opioid receptors in the body as poppy-based opioids, and its overall effects are much less dangerous. Evidence strongly supports the idea that, while addiction to mitragyna is possible, the addiction and withdrawal symptoms have proven to be on par with that of caffeine addiction. Mitragyna is frequently used to lessen the symptoms of opiate withdrawal by providing the same level of pain relief as opiates, without the damaging effects of the opiates on all of the organs of the body. Further, when using mitragyna to help break the cycle of opiate addiction, mitragyna provides many other valuable properties.

Independent studies on alkaloids found in mitragyna leaves have shown that it strengthens and improves the overall function of the immune system. Mitragyna leaf exhibits free-radical scavenging and antimicrobial activity, and is naturally high in antioxidants. Besides aiding the immune system in repairing damage done to the body from opioids, mitragyna can be used to help fight everything from the common cold to cancer.

Mitragyna also works by optimizing certain metabolic processes and impacting hormone levels. This ability accounts for its usefulness in treating anxiety, depression, PTSD, regulating blood pressure, increasing energy, regulating blood sugar, and suppressing the appetite. Increased circulation and the ability of mitragyna leaves to deliver larger amounts of oxygen to the blood help boost energy and increase libido. In a society that is becoming increasingly dependent on antidepressants, energy drinks and questionable appetite-suppressing drugs, mitragyna, with its lack of long-term side effects, provides an effective, valuable alternative.

Mitragyna, while being useful for many different conditions, is dependent on proper dosage and personal tolerance levels, which is where problems often arise. Mitragyna should always be used under the supervision and direction of a Certified Herbalist or health care professional, especially if you are taking any other medications or have known health-issues.

Purchasing mitragyna can be a challenge. Finding a reputable source is important, as much of what is currently on the market at gas stations and convenience stores may contain contaminants or other ingredients, as do many of the online sources. Reputable companies to purchase from will clearly state how and from where the mitragyna was obtained, what strain it belongs to, and if any other ingredients were added to it.

Mitragyna is available as a capsule, a powdered or crushed leaf, or an extract. The capsule form is the most popular, but the powder is the most effective form, especially when taken as a tea. Others take 1/2 teaspoon of crushed leaf in applesauce. The extract is not recommended due to the variable concentration that may result in a higher than recommended dosage.

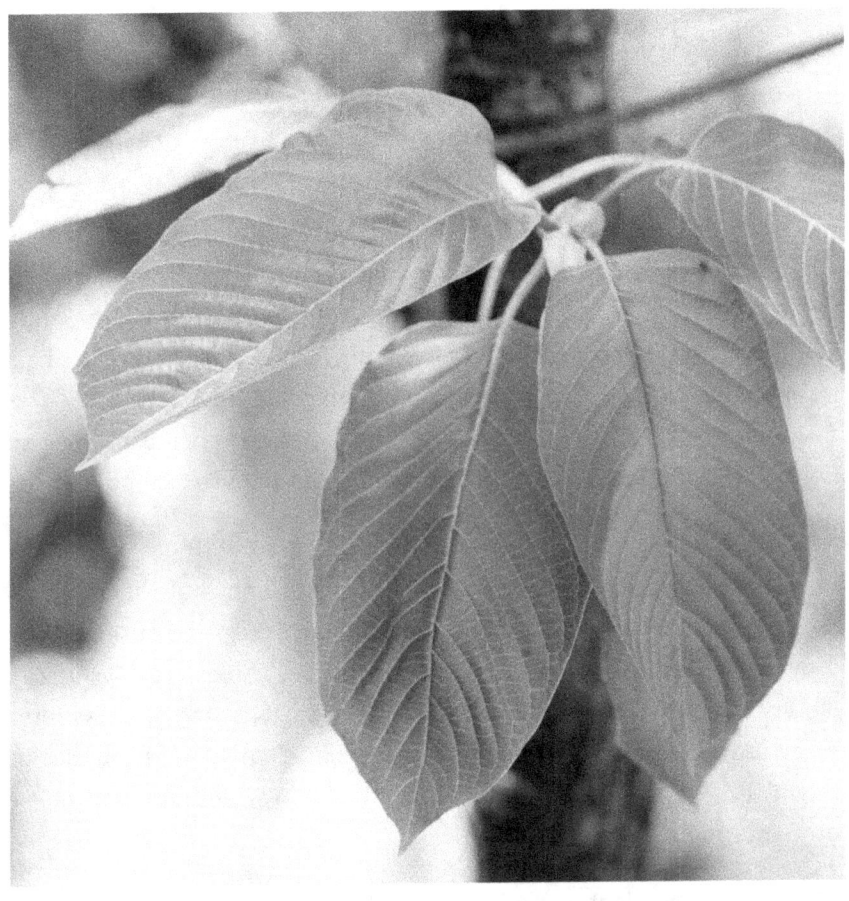

Mitragyna speciosa. Photo courtesy of the National Center for Complementary and Integrative Health - NIH

70 ARROWROOT : GLUTEN-FREE FLOUR SUBSTITUTE AND MORE

Arrowroot is not a native Missouri plant, but it can be grown here and was commercially cultivated in Georgia and South Carolina in the early 1800's. It likes the more tropical areas, and was introduced to South Florida in the 19th century, where it is thought the Seminole Indians had a role in developing it as a food source. An underused food crop, the rhizomes are an excellent source of starch that can be substituted for flour. The plant gets its name from its centuries old use as a poultice to draw poison from wounds.

Arrowroot powder is considered an excellent carbohydrate source, and the roots contain 25 – 30% starch. Nutritionally, 100 grams of Arrowroot provides 65 calories, 4.24 g of carbohydrates, 0 cholesterol, 1.3 gm of dietary fiber, 26 mg of sodium and an whopping 454 mg of potassium. Arrowroot is also an excellent source of niacin, pyridoxine, riboflavin, thiamine, Vitamin A, Vitamin C, Calcium, Iron, Magnesium, and many other nutrients.

Medicinally, the plant is used as a demulcent (like mucinex to break up phlegm), and for its anti-diarrhea effects. It also has benefits as a urinary antiseptic, and helps to lower cholesterol. It may also have pro-biotic properties. Arrowroot reduces inflammation, and is also an antiseptic, making it a good choice to treat external wounds and skin lesions.

As a food, arrowroot is most often consumed in the form of baked goods and jellies. Substituting arrowroot makes a perfectly clear fruit gel, unlike cornstarch that can clump and make the sauce cloudy. It also prevents ice crystals in homemade ice cream. Arrowroot is gluten free with twice the thickening power of wheat flour due to its pectin content. Arrowroot products can be frozen, unlike cornstarch that breaks down with the freezing and thawing process. When making salmon patties, zucchini fritters or meat loaf, arrowroot is an excellent binding agent, holding the mixture together during cooking.

There are several studies comparing the texture of arrowroot, and the way it feels in your mouth, to products made with flour. In one study, it was found that arrowroot enhanced the buttery taste in baked products, and the testers found the very fine texture of the products made with arrowroot had a melt in the mouth texture as compared with the grittier texture of flour-based products. Starch from the plant is easily digested, and is safe for infants, persons in ill health, and those with wheat allergies.

Growing and processing Arrowroot

Extracting the starch is a simple procedure, which can be done at home. Those that make their living from wild harvesting often add arrowroot powder to their product offerings.

When growing arrowroot, spacing the plants about 16 inches apart and 10 inches deep gives a higher yield on the number and weight of the tubers per plant. Once you harvest the roots, clean and wash them thoroughly, then grate them into a fine pulp. Strain the pulp through a fine strainer or cheesecloth into a container, using a little water as needed. Let the sediment settle, then carefully pour off the fluid, letting the fine powder left behind dry. Some people wash and strain the pulp 3 times to get the whitest powder possible. Dry the processed starch in a solar dryer or other method at 45 degrees for six hours, then sifting through a flour sifter if there are any large clumps. The resulting arrowroot powder can then be substituted for flour in recipes, added to soups, or used in making jellies.

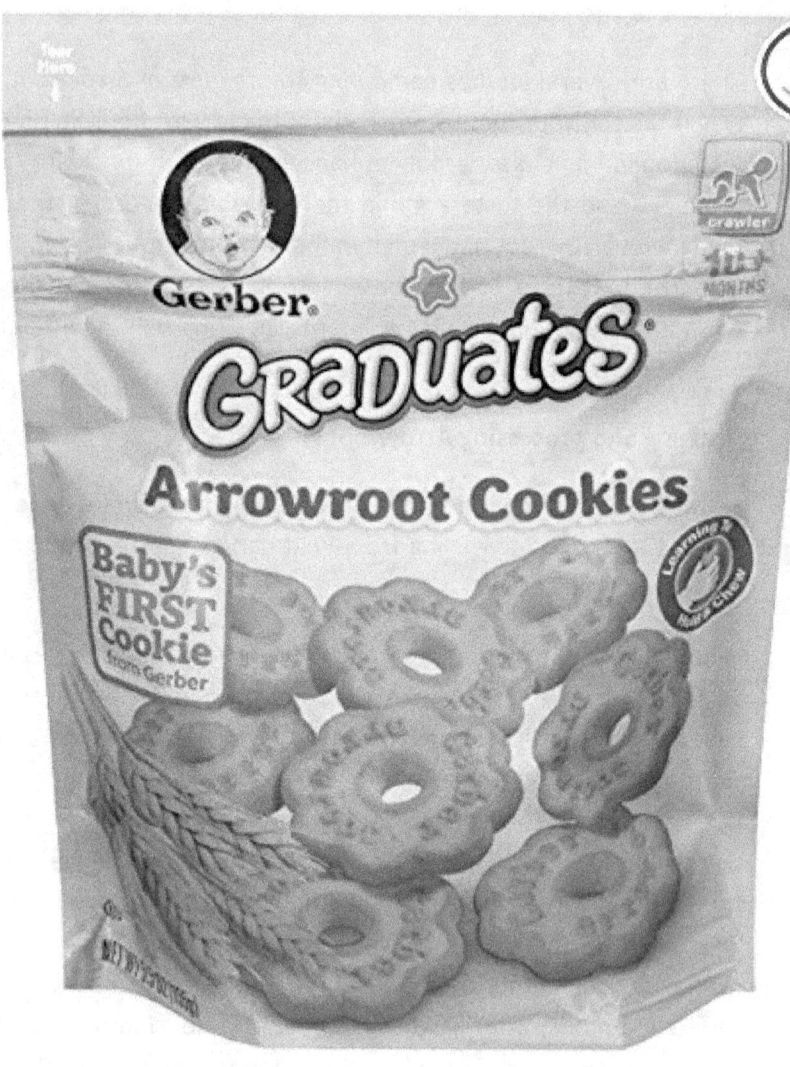

Arrowroot cookies are popular for babies in many parts of the world.

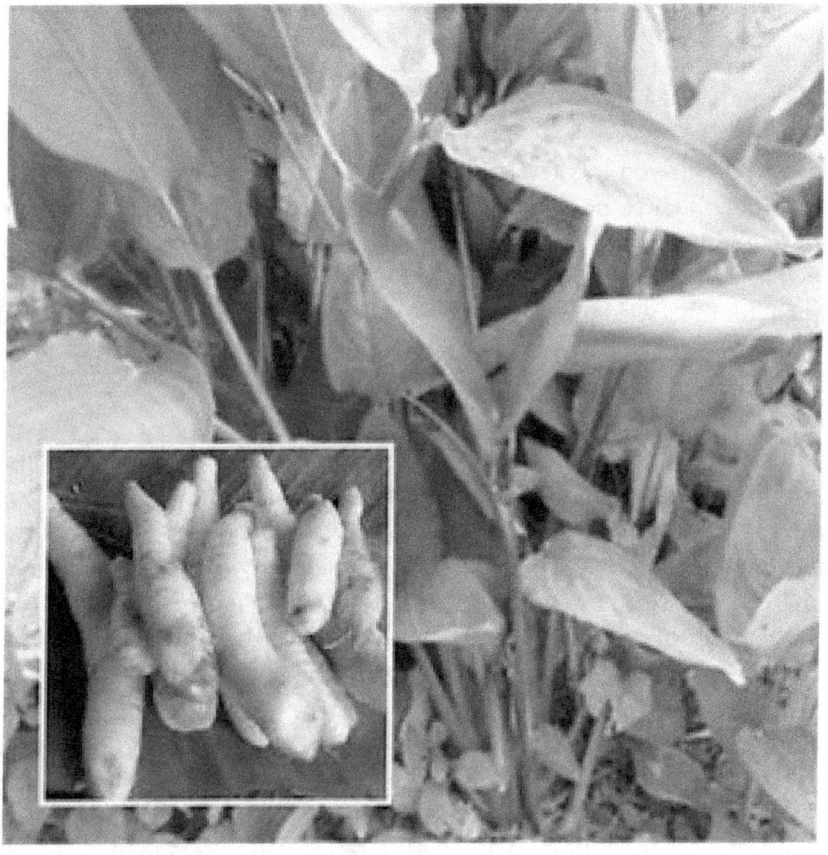

The tubers of the arrowroot plant have both medicinal and nutritional value.

72 SPRING HERB WALK

By: Tamara Glascock

Spring has arrived in the Ozarks, bringing with it some crazy weather and an abundance of weeds and flowers just waiting to be plucked and put to good use. Our grandparents and great-grandparents knew exactly what to do with all of those beautiful spring greens popping up, but much of that wisdom has been lost along the way. Local Herbalist Tamara Glascock is attempting to bring that knowledge back and share it with others in our community.

Last Saturday, Tamara hosted a Spring Herb Walk at her Edgar Springs farm, Tranquil Haven Hollow. Armed with packets of information on useful herbs, guests were led around the property as she pointed out native edible and medicinal plants, how to identify them, and explained how to prepare many of them. "We have forgotten how to use what Mother Nature gives us," Tamara stated. "I want to teach people how to make the most of what the land can provide in terms of food and medicine. This time of year, many people are heading outdoors armed with herbicides and lawn mowers to kill off some of the most useful plants like dandelions, shepherd's purse and burdock. I want to show people how to harvest them, prepare them, and use them to keep themselves a bit healthier. I would love to see more people encouraging them to grow rather than trying to kill them off. Many of them make lovely additions to flower beds and gardens!"

As she led the herb walk, Tamara did exactly that. The walk, which lasted just under an hour, was filled with information on what many of the native plants are used for. Dandelion and chickweed were everywhere, and she explained how adding them to a salad or making a tea of the fresh leaves and flowers helped clear the body of all the toxins that tend to build up in our system over the cold winter months when it is more difficult to obtain fresh produce, or get outside for a bit of fresh air and sunshine. She showed how simple it was to grab a handful and make a delicious 'lawn salad', or a cup of tea. Many of the guests were happy to pluck leaves to taste as they made their way from plant to plant.

The walk was followed by a casual question and answer session while guests sipped tea and munched on a salad filled with freshly-picked leaves of lemon balm, plantain, yellow dock leaves and other common 'weeds' that were gathered by guests during the walk.

Spring isn't the only time to find medicinal herbs growing in the area, though. Throughout the summer and well into the fall, the Ozarks has so much to offer. When asked about some of the weeds popping up that were a bit more difficult to identify right now, Tamara revealed that she will be hosting herb walks throughout the year, as well as classes on the variety of ways to use herbs and plants. "There are many herbs like mullein, burdock and yarrow that are incredibly valuable in terms of food and medicine, but, until they start to bloom, they can be easy to overlook. I will be putting together another herb walk in the fall when these plants are close to being ready to harvest."

You can contact Tamara Glascock at tamarasherbes@yahoo.com or call 573-612-9213.

Photos by Becky Duell.

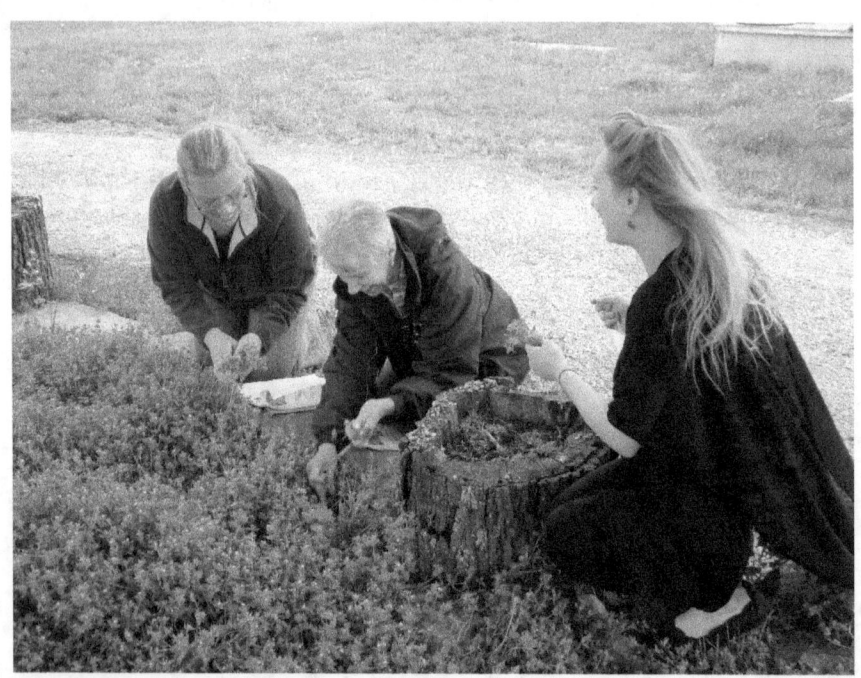

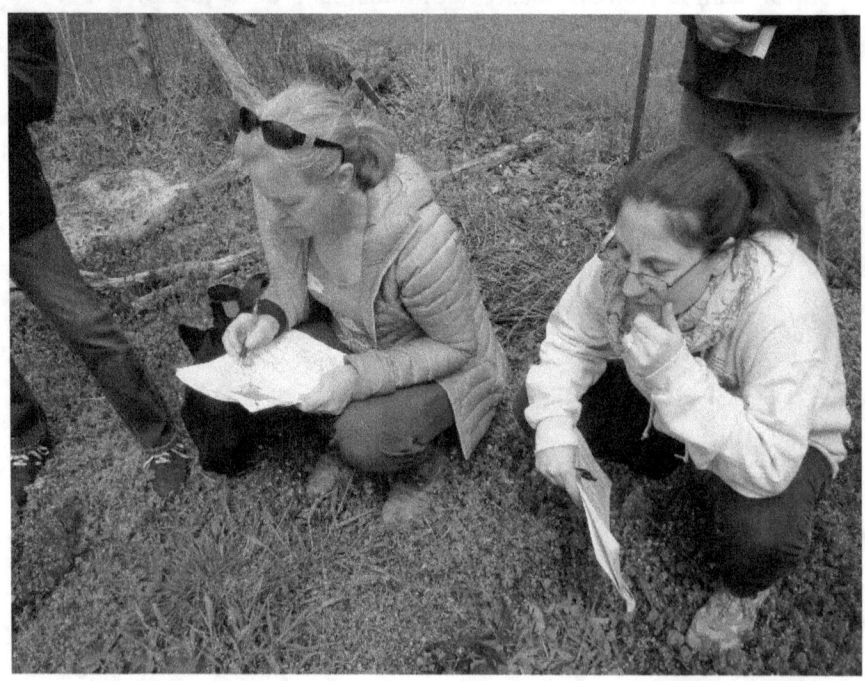

72 THE BIG FAT LIE

Many of us remember the vilification of eggs and butter as we were growing up. Crisco and margarine were offered as a healthy alternative to butter, and "Egg Beaters" replaced whole eggs, but certainly never beat them.

Guess what? Since the USDA first recommended a low-fat diet in 1980, obesity rates in the U.S. have risen dramatically. The new USDA guidelines in the form of "My Plate" have completely eliminated the essential category of fats and oils.

The idea that saturated fats are unhealthy was first planted in our brain in the 1950's, when a researcher named Ancel Keys conducted a series of flawed studies and ended up on the board of the American Heart Association, a new organization launched by Proctor and Gamble – maker of Crisco. In the early sixties, Keys himself found that no matter how much cholesterol research subjects ate, their blood levels stayed the same; even in people consuming up to 3.000 mg per day. In comparison, one large egg has 200 mg of cholesterol. In fact, eating 2 – 3 eggs a day for years has no more than a minimal effect on cholesterol. Despite the contradictory facts, Keys persisted in manipulating public opinion, promoting Crisco as a healthy alternative.

Sugar, rather than cholesterol, is the food most closely associated with death due to a coronary event. It's also the entity most closely correlated with tooth decay, not an absence of fluoride, as some would have you believe.

Low cholesterol levels have an association with cancer. As everyone in the country went on low cholesterol diets, the incidence of cancer went up. In 1981, there were almost a dozen human studies showing the link between lowered cholesterol and cancer, especially colon cancer; in fact men with cholesterol levels lower than 190 mg/dl were three times more like to get colon cancer than men with levels higher than 220 mg/dl.

In 1992, an expert panel reviewed all the heart disease data on women and found that those with low cholesterol had higher mortality rates. In response to the evidence, most European nations, including Great Britain, no longer recommend limiting cholesterol intake. In the United States, however, the cholesterol "limit" is capped at 300 mg day (1.5 eggs.) and the myriad of cholesterol-free items on the grocery shelves subtly remind shoppers that cholesterol is the enemy. In fact, replacing animal fats with vegetable fats has no effect on serum cholesterol.

Total cholesterol is made up of HDL, high density or "good" cholesterol, and LDL, low density or "bad" cholesterol. LDL goes up with obesity, smoking, high blood pressure and no exercise, while HDL rises with a healthier life-style. Guess what raises HDL levels the most? Eating saturated fat, which is the ONLY food known to do so.

Triglyceride levels also play a role, and it turns out total cholesterol is NOT a good predictor of health risk, but levels of HDL cholesterol are, with levels below 36 mg/dl correlated with an 8 times higher risk of heart attack. Drug companies tried, but failed, to find a way to raise HDL, but found they could lower LDL levels with drugs, thus the billion-dollar world of statin drugs was born.

Fat doesn't make you fat.

The most likely hormone causing obesity is insulin, which is triggered with eating carbohydrates. On the other hand, consuming fat is the least likely to cause weight gain, as it is the only macronutrient that does not stimulate insulin reduction. With more and more people eating low fat diets and scrupulously avoiding cholesterol, obesity continues to rise and cardiac events remain the leading cause of death in the United States.

74 THE BERRIES OF MISSOURI

Did you know that there are six varieties of edible berries native to Missouri? Yes, it is true, and all of them can be found in our area. Mark your calendar now for the best time to harvest.

Gooseberries

Gooseberry plants are found all over Missouri, and provide the earliest fruit for berry pickers. The end of May and early June is when the fruit appears, and is picked when it reaches about one quarter inch in size. They are VERY tart and require a lot of sugar to make them palatable, but a lot of folks love them and they are also very high in vitamin C. The berries are generally green to light yellow, turning dark purple when they are fully ripe. Gooseberries can have a fungus that kills white pines, and they are banned in some states. Make sure they don't grow within 1500 feet of your white pine trees.

Blackberries

All Missourians are familiar with the native blackberry. During the Great Depression, it was a staple as well as a treat that supplemented many a meal during those lean days. Missouri has several species of blackberries, and the best time to harvest is typically in July. How moist they are depends on the rainfall, with some years certainly better than others. Often those growing close to the ground, and hardest to pick, are the juiciest.

Raspberry

My favorite berry of all, I thought Missouri raspberries were a myth until 3 years ago when I found a huge patch behind the workshop. In addition to being delicious, and exceedingly easy to turn into jam due to the high pectin content, wild raspberries protect against ulcerative colitis and several kinds of cancer. When making jam, be sure to retain the seeds, as they are part of what makes this berry a super food! The plant blooms with clusters of white flowers as early as April in most years, but will likely be late this year due to the delayed growing season. Unlike the red raspberries we are familiar with, Missouri wild raspberries are blue/black when ripe. They can be distinguished from blackberries because raspberries don't have a white core like blackberries, and they also have a hollow indentation at the top that allows them to pop right off the stem when picked. Raspberry thickets get larger every year as they re-root themselves. Be on the lookout, or the wild turkeys will beat you to the fruit!

Wild Strawberries

Wild strawberries are found throughout Missouri, and the native species is a parent to the commercial strawberry that you find in the grocery store. The plant is easy to spot, and looks like a typical strawberry plant with white flowers in clusters with five white petals that bloom from April to May (so now is the time to look). The leaves are dark green, in groups of three, with toothed lobes and hairy stems. The small berries are about 1/2 inch in diameter, and ripen in June and July. Rumors about wild strawberry being poisonous are not true, but there is a "mock strawberry" out there, also called Indian strawberry, that has yellow petals and tasteless fruit. Missouri wild strawberries are reportedly the favorite food of box turtles.

Blueberries

Three species of wild blueberry are found in Missouri, with a long season that extends from April through September. The low bush blueberry is considered the tastiest. The shrub grows from 1 to 3 feet tall in central and southern Missouri, and the fruit ripens over the summer month to a deep blue color. Most folks pick immediately as the berries become ripe, freezing them until quantities allow making blueberry muffins, pancakes, syrup or jam.

Dewberries

Missouri has several varieties of Dewberry. They look like blackberries, but produce their fruit a little earlier, beginning in June. In addition, instead of growing on a small shrub like a blackberry plant, dewberries are low to the ground with trailing vines that catch your pants as you are walking through a field. They are used and eaten just like the blackberry.

It is hard to imagine anywhere else on earth with as many edible native berries as can be found right here in the Ozarks. Pretty much everything you need to make a mixed berry pie!

74 THE "WHAT IFS" AND WARNING SIGNS

My husband passed away on May 14. One week after our tenth anniversary, he seemed to be the picture of health. One month prior, our home was badly damaged by a F-1 tornado. An independent man, he was doing most of the work himself, pushing hard to finish by the end of May. He worked many 18 hour days.

Four days prior to his death, he told me he had passed a kidney stone. He vomited quite a bit that day, and said lying on the heating pad "saved my life." He has had at least 3 bouts of kidney stone issues, so it wasn't too unusual. I keep testing strips, which have been discussed in this column before, and had him test his urine. Strangely, there was no microscopic blood. Unusual, and I should have investigated further, but he said he was feeling fine now.

He continued to work hard all weekend, spending hours painting the ceilings and walls, ordered lots of building supplies, and had them delivered for an Amish work crew coming to help on Tuesday. He had a strenuous day on Monday, harvesting the logs from the trees that had been felled during the tornado, taking them to the sawmill. The friend who helped him later told me he seemed fine, but "there were a few things that went wrong, but we fixed them and it didn't seem to bother him." He completed some wiring in the house, and stacked the supplies for the building crew coming the following morning. That evening, he went to Houston to conduct a training session for the Missouri Defense Force, grabbing a quick meal from Hardees, and his only vice, a large Mountain Dew.

During the meeting, the men attending noticed he was taking a lot of deep breaths, and dropping his head, but he seemed fine and never complained. They thought possibly he had indigestion.

When he arrived home about 9 pm, an unexpected rainstorm had popped up, so he raced around covering the building supplies with tarps. He came back in the house, talking normally, when he took a huge breath, like a sigh, and collapsed to the floor. Immediate CPR was unsuccessful, and when paramedics arrived, there was no cardiac activity on the monitor. Our best and prolonged efforts could not bring him back.

So where did things go so wrong? How can a 46-year-old man just die without warning? The fact is, there were lots of warning signs, and I don't want anyone to miss them as both Brad and I did.

Let's start with Mountain Dew. As coroner, last year I pronounced a young man, Brad's age with "caffeine-induced cardiac event causing a probable arrhythmia." He was surrounded with cans of Mountain Dew, and toxicology showed an extremely high caffeine level. An overdose of caffeine may cause rapid or irregular heartbeat and breathing trouble. In rare cases, caffeine overdose can result in death due to convulsions or irregular heartbeat. Brad was drinking large quantities of Mountain Dew a day, as he was keeping up his energy on all the work to be done.

As I look back, I think the supposed kidney stone the week before was likely a smaller heart attack. Many, many times before a heart attack men will say "it's just indigestion." Guess what? Indigestion should be taken seriously. Definitely worth getting vital signs with a home blood pressure monitor, and counting pulse rate and checking to see if it is regular. Any irregularities in heart rate, especially associated with indigestion, warrant a trip to the doctor, or even emergency room.

You won't always have chest pain with a heart attack. It is common to have tooth and jaw pain, even back pain, although the most common is left arm pain. My husband's main symptom, looking back, was shortness of breath that had nothing to do with his lungs. Even a mild heart attack can affect the electrical activity of the heart. The heart has to beat in perfect synchrony to deliver oxygen to all the cells, without that, you become air hungry. I suspect this is what happened to Brad. A simple EKG will show if the heart isn't working properly, and can even tell you if you've had a mild heart attack in the past.

This is my message: Concentrated caffeine drinks like Mountain Dew are dangerous and addictive. Even more importantly, our stoic, strong husbands will likely deny anything is wrong. Do whatever you have to do, and MAKE them seek some sort of medical attention when symptoms start. For me, the saddest death is a preventable one.

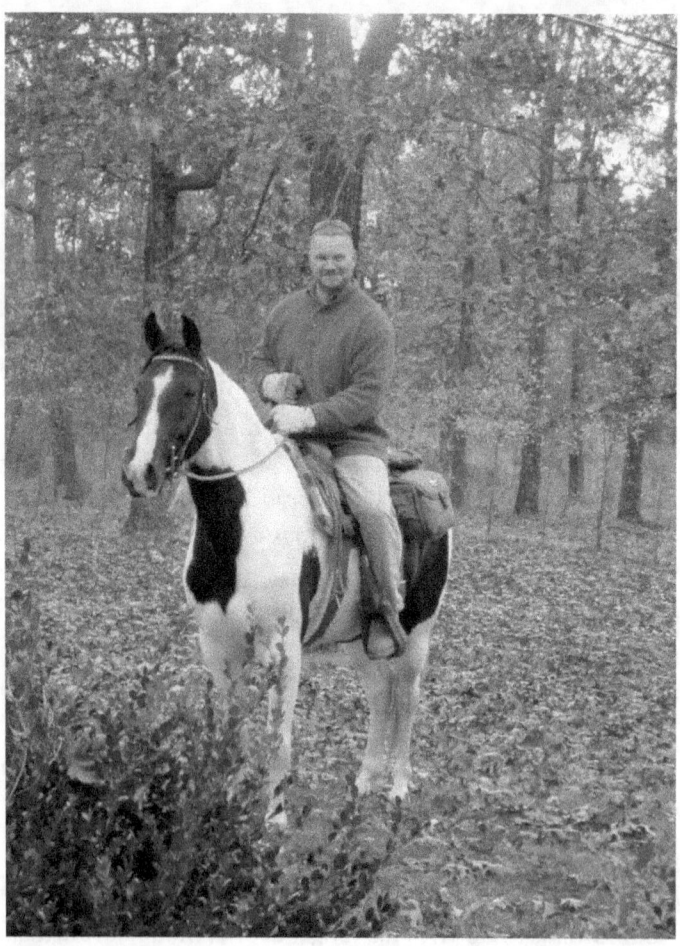

Bradley Vincent North

75 PAIN

By: Tamara Glascock

Occasionally, we all experience pain. Headaches, backaches, injuries, or life cause us to head to the medicine cabinet for a dose of ibuprofen or acetaminophen. Unfortunately, those options come with a fair amount of danger.

Each year, acetaminophen overdose is responsible for more than 56,000 emergency room visits, 2,600 hospitalizations, and an estimated 458 deaths due to acute liver failure. It is also linked to severe, sometimes fatal, skin diseases, including Stevens-Johnson Syndrome (SJS), Toxic Epidermal Necrolysis (TENS), and Acute Generalized Exanthematous Pustulosis (AGEP).

Ibuprofen is responsible for just as many side effects, including nausea, vomiting, headache, rash, heartburn, dermatitis, decreased white blood cells, red blood cells, and platelets, and acute renal failure. So, what is a person to do to get a bit of relief when your level of pain is too much to bear, but you don't want to risk these side effects, or head to the doctor for something even more dangerous than ibuprofen or acetaminophen? Fortunately, there are many natural options that provide profound relief without the risk of destroying your body.

Willow bark, the precursor to aspirin, contains the chemical salicin. Salicin is a potent pain killer, anti-inflammatory, and fever reducer. It is especially useful for relieving headaches and back pain, which are often the result of internal inflammation. Chewing on a small piece of willow bark is the traditional way to take it, but it can also be powdered and placed in a capsule, taken as an extract, or made into soothing cup of hot tea. While there have been a limited number of reports that willow bark caused an upset stomach, it is considered extremely safe and effective for pain relief.

Capsaicin, an ingredient found in hot chili peppers, is an antioxidant and anti-inflammatory. It also known to help desensitize the pain receptors over time, providing relief from chronic pain. It can often be found in topical creams for joint and muscle aches, and works by drawing blood to the surface, which speeds the healing of strained or damaged muscles. While many people mistakenly believe that hot peppers cause stomach issues, in truth, capsaicin has been shown to soothe and heal ulcers and other digestive issues.

Ginger, and its close relation turmeric, both common kitchen spices, and are both powerful anti-inflammatories that are especially useful in relieving pain associated with arthritis. They contain a wealth of antioxidants that break down existing inflammation and acidity in the fluid in the joints. Adding a bit of ginger or turmeric to your food is a wonderful way to take them, but they can also be taken dried or made into a delicious cup of tea!

Wild lettuce, also called wild opium lettuce, is an ancient pain remedy that has been forgotten by most people, but has recently been the focus of many medical studies. It grows freely throughout the Ozarks, and is often mistaken for a common weed. Its ability to relieve pain is on par with that of mitragyna speciosa (kratom), and works in much the same way. Both act on the system as an opioid, without the risk of addiction. Wild lettuce contains lactones, a substance that acts on the central nervous system to calm the nerves, which cause pain sensations.

So, the next time you are seeking a bit of relief from pain, head to your kitchen or front yard instead of the medicine cabinet. Whether it is a simple headache or chronic pain, finding relief doesn't have to come with the fear of dangerous, long-term side effects.

76 CLUTTER, SANITY AND THE MINIMALIST MOVEMENT

How many have ever said, "When my house is a mess, I'm a mess?" For hoarders, clutter and trash bring comfort and security. For most of us, watching an episode of Hoarders is likely to bring on a cleaning spree.

Why do we crave organization? It's the way we are constructed at the cellular level. Our body is made up of millions of tissues, cells and biological systems that are extremely organized. When no longer organized, as with the disruption or cancer or other diseases, our system suffers. We even have a circadian rhythm, with regular cycles for eating, sleeping, hormone releases and elimination, to name a few. Just like the affect internal organization has on our life, external organization has an impact as well, and is easier to manage.

Having too much stuff leads to anxiety. In one study conducted by the University of California, cortisol, the stress hormone, was measured in 30 couples. Women with messy homes had higher levels of cortisol, and reported feeling more stressed. Men did not seem to have the same reaction to clutter. A 2010 study looked at the way 60 women discussed their homes. Those who said their homes were "cluttered" or full of "unfinished projects" were more likely to be depressed and fatigued than women who described their homes as "restful" and "restorative." Once again, women with messy homes had higher levels of cortisol.

It is a paradox of life that the more stuff we have, the less joy we feel. I think every reader can think back to a time when they were really struggling, but making it by on a shoestring; reusing, recycling, repurposing. Hindsight is 20/20, but most of us have happy memories of those days.

Dozens of studies have compared those in "minimalist" homes with those that are cluttered. There is clearly an inverse relationship between too much clutter and your psychological health. Clutter can actually sap your energy, making it hard to clean up the mess that is causing distress in the first place! A 2011 study found that clutter makes difficult to focus on a particular task due to the fact the visual cortex can be overwhelmed by task-irrelevant objects, districting attention, and destroying efficiency.

So how did our house get is such a mess? We tend to accumulate items we think we might need in the future. The problem is these non-essentials take up space that could be better used by more necessary things. Because of the emotional attachment we can have, sometimes donating items helps to let go. For some things, taking a photo is all that is needed to release the physical item; for example, scan old documents and photos to disk.

Time is in short supply for everyone. Try each day to organize and clean not a whole room, but rather a space. Always have a donation box open and ready to receive unnecessary items. Regarding clothing, a good rule of thumb is that if you haven't worn it once in the past year, you never will again. Some experts recommend reducing your wardrobe to 33 items or less. In college, I had a psychology professor who owned only two outfits that she rotated. She was one of the most amazing people I've ever met, with a brilliant mind and uncluttered with "stuff."

Above all, owing less is spiritually healthy. The Bible cautions us not to worship objects, and to share what we have with those less fortunate. As a deadly sin, hanging onto clutter can be considered a form of gluttony. Strive to be a clean, lean servant of the Lord.

77 NATURAL COSMETICS

By: Candice Schwien

We as women tend to enhance our natural beauty by wearing cosmetics. Sometimes it can be very difficult to find high quality makeup that fits our skin tone exactly. There are also times when we find just the right color and take it home, only to have a reaction to it the first time we use it. I have fairly sensitive skin, so for years I tried to find makeup that worked with my skin and eventually stopped wasting money on products that only caused pain.

However, after my son was born I knew I needed to start trying to find cosmetics again. (You moms out there will know what I mean when I say those sleepless nights are cause to find great concealer for circles under the eyes.) A beautiful person in my life stepped in and helped me get started. From there I have tried to find ways to create healthier options, and less expensive ones.

Did you know?

The word cosmetic comes from the Greek word kosmeticos, which means "skilled at adornment."

Making your own cosmetics is perfect if you want to use ingredients that are good for you and the environment. It's also a great choice if you struggle to match your skin tone and type, and if you suffer from allergies. You can experiment with the recipes and change them up depending on colors and densities. It does not matter what kind of cosmetics you use. ALWAYS remember to wash them off at night. Did you know leaving cosmetics on overnight can age your skin by breaking it down? Here is a great evening cleanser that is great for all skin types.

Evening Cleanser

1/4 cup jojoba oil
1/2 teaspoon vitamin E oil
3 drops lavender oil

Mix all together. Apply to the face and wipe it off with clean cotton balls. Not only does this remove the makeup, but it also moisturizes the skin for the evening.

Sweet Almond Facial Cream

2 teaspoons non-petroleum jelly
2 teaspoons cocoa butter
2 Tablespoons sweet almond oil (Jojoba/hazelnut can also be used)
2 drops chamomile calendula or lavender essential oil

Warm the non-petroleum jelly, cocoa butter and sweet almond oil over low heat until the cocoa butter has melted. Remove from heat and cool while stirring the blend occasionally. Add essential oil and mix well. Store in an airtight container. Apply to the face and lips before going outside. (Works best in colder temperatures.)

Healing Lip Balm

2 Tablespoons bees wax
1/2 cup jojoba oil
1 teaspoon honey
1 teaspoon aloe vera gel
10 drops tea tree essential oil
(a few drops of your favorite essential oil)

Melt the beeswax over low heat. Add the jojoba oil, honey, aloe vera gel, and tea tree essential oil. Warm and then remove from heat. Stir rapidly with a whisk until cool. Add your favorite flavor of essential oil. Coconut oil, wintergreen, clove, peppermint, or lavender are popular choices. Pour the balm into small containers, baby food jars or reused chapstick containers work well. Apply to the lips to help prevent or health chapping, cracking, and/or blisters.

Beautiful Facial Powder

1/2 cup fine white cosmetic clay
1 Tablespoon powdered rose petals
1 Tablespoon powdered walnut hulls
* For medium to fair skin, mix the cosmetic clay with the rose petals.
* For medium to dark skin, mix the cosmetic clay with the walnut hulls.

Apply the mixture lightly with a fluff brush or a cotton ball to set makeup. Or use it throughout the day to absorb oil on the forehead, nose and chin.

Tips

Always treat facial skin very gently. Especially around the eyes.
Apply creams and cleansers with light dabs.
Use soft facial tissues or cotton balls. Never use paper towels, toilet tissue, or rough pads.
Avoid hard scrubbing when removing makeup.
When applying lip balm, never stretch your lips; this highlights fine lines and wrinkles.

Bonus

Jojoba oil is a great eye moisturizer at nighttime. Simply dab the oil around the eyes with your finger. Remember to avoid the lashes and lids.

Place a cold tea bag over each eye to relieve puffy and tired eyes. Rest for 15 minutes.

If your eyes are strained, dip cotton balls in a mixture of cold witch hazel, milk, or tea and apply to the eyes for 15 minutes.

For more tips and ideas from Candice, find her on Facebook/Natural Country Health.

78 MULBERRIES

Following my article last month entitled Berries of Missouri, it was brought to my attention by an attentive reader that I had left out what is possibly the most important berry of all, the mulberry.

You may be surprised to know that the mulberry plant is most prized in other countries, not as a food, but as silkworm feed and animal fodder. Here in Missouri, the mulberry is a very hardy and fast-growing plant. I have a terrific mulberry tree on my place that a horse chewed down to the ground on not one, but two occasions, and is currently 6 feet tall and loaded with berries. They have a very strong root system, with roots forming a dense tangle in the soil, preventing erosion and keeping the tree stable.

Silk made from the mulberry plant accounts for 90% of silk production globally. A protein contained in the leaves is used to feed silkworms, who convert it into silk protein that is made into silk yarn. As livestock fodder, mulberry makes excellent animal feed, with nutrients of sodium, calcium and phosphorus. One study showed an increase in milk production in cows fed with mulberry leaf stalks. On poultry farms, mulberry leaf meal has resulted in greater egg production. Horses apparently love it.

People love mulberries too! The fruit of the mulberry is used to make wine, jam and soft drinks, and contains amino acids, vitamins and important minerals. Making mulberry jam is a snap because of the naturally high pectin content, and it jells easily. Mulberry juice can be used for both coloring and flavoring; add some juice to your white cake batter for a unique version of a red velvet cake.

Medicinal Uses

In some countries, mulberry is considered a sacred plant due to its medicinal uses, including improvement of eyesight, protecting the liver, controlling diabetes, and facilitating weight loss.

In addition to the medicinal uses mentioned above, there are numerous studies documenting the antioxidant, antiviral (including HIV), anti-inflammatory, anti-allergy, lipid lowering and neuro protective properties of the mulberry. The leaves have chemicals that are have been found to lower both blood pressure and cholesterol levels in humans. Compared to other berry producing plants, mulberry leaf extract is most effective in lowering iron levels.

The studies that have been done on the effect of mulberry on lowering blood pressure have looked only at white mulberry (the native Missouri Mulberry is the red variety). The results show that white mulberry acts by relaxing the blood vessels so the heart does not have to pump as hard, resulting in lowered blood pressure, equally as effective as the drug Verapamil.

One component of the mulberry leaf, fagomine, can help stimulate insulin secretion in pancreatic islet cells; lowering blood glucose levels. Animal studies have also shown that mulberry leaf extract also has an anti-obesity action in laboratory animals.

It is thought that amyloid plaques in the brain (think sticky tangles), are at least one cause of Alzheimer's disease. Mulberry leaf contains compounds that prevent the formation of these plaques.

Environment protectors

1 mulberry tree can remove 4162 kg of carbon dioxide out of the air and replace it with 3064 kg of oxygen. Mulberry trees can also absorb heavy metals in the soil, making them valuable in hazmat clean up areas by removing lead, cadmium, and copper from the soil.

If you'd like to have a mulberry tree, or two, on your place, native seedlings are available at the George O. White Nursery on Shafer Rd.

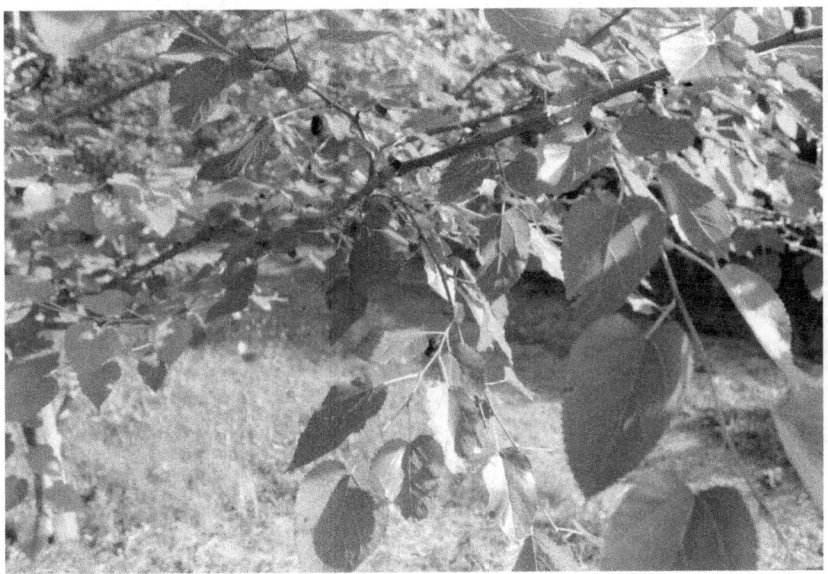

My mulberry tree is heavily laden with berries, despite heavy prunings by my horse.

80 ECHINACEA

As I was leaving the 25th Anniversary party of the Roby Lions Club last weekend, I spotted large patches of Echinacea – coneflower – growing alongside the highway on Hwy. 17. To those who saw me in the ditch, I was taking pictures and gathering a few seeds.

Our native coneflowers belong to the Echinacea species, only native to Canada and the United States. They are coveted plants, used to support the immune system, warding off respiratory ailments like the common cold and treating upper respiratory symptoms caused by bacterial infections. The plant has been a staple in the natural cures arsenal since the 1950's, and is very safe to use, with the exception of a rare allergic reaction. There are no documented drug/herb interactions associated with Echinacea. Lewis and Clark learned about the plant from the Native Americans during their Expedition in the early 1800's, and even went to the trouble to send some plants to President Jefferson because of the plant's importance.

While we think of Echinacea as a treatment for the common cold, it is also useful in wound healing and other applications. 19 Native American tribes are documented as using coneflower as a source of Echinacea to treat not only coughs and colds, but also treatment of mumps, as a mouth disinfectant, a painkiller for a head and stomach ache, and as snakebite treatment. There are also reports of Echinacea being used to treat urinary tract infections (similar to Goldenseal) and to prevent herpes outbreaks. Active ingredients found in the plant include caffeic acid, essential oils, polysaccharides, polyacetylene and flavonoids, to name a few.

There are nine distinct native Echinacea species, and in our abundant Ozarks, we can find five of those. The Glade coneflower variety is found mostly in the eastern Ozarks. William Clark, of the Lewis and Clark expedition, famously wrote about the narrow-leaved purple coneflower *Echinacea angustifolia*, "I collected a Plant the root of which is a Cure for the Bite of a mad dog & Snake which I shall Send..." Pale purple coneflower is the most widespread in Missouri. Yellow coneflower resembles a black eyed Susan with deep brown centers and yellow rays. Narrow leaf coneflower is thought to have been introduced to our state, but grows naturally in Iowa, Nebraska and Kansas.

Poaching and sustainability

Because of the inherent value of the coneflower, it is subject to poaching, and there are laws restricting digging it up but the roadside and other places it grows wild. It is hard, if not impossible to transplant, so root digging is generally associated with plant poaching in order to profit from sale of the root. Even without laws, Echinacea should never been dug up by the root in its native habitat; instead collect a few seeds to easily grow your own in your home garden. It takes only two years to bloom from seed, and as a perennial, it will come back year after year. Growing Echinacea commercially to meet the popular demand for the product, sparing native plants, is currently under economic consideration.

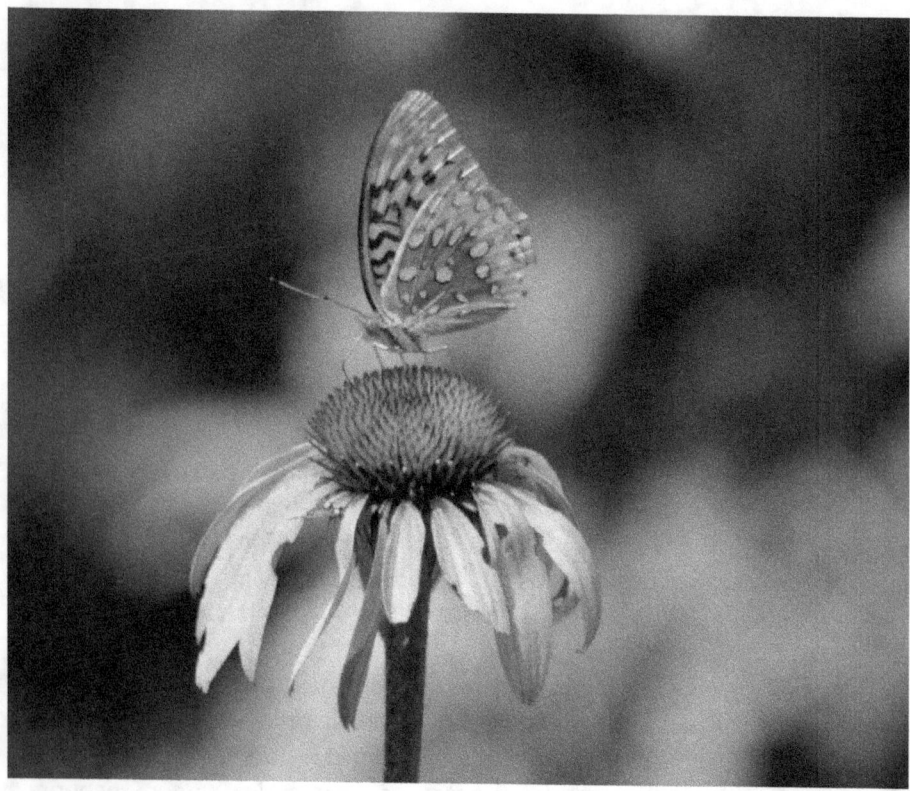

Native coneflowers are important not only as a medicinal plant, but also help the environment. As this photo captured by Rick Mansfield beautifully illustrates, they also provide nectar for Monarch butterflies. Many birds feed on the abundant seeds, and the plant itself prevents erosion.

80 TREATING COMMON AILMENTS

By Tamara Glascock

Getting sick is never fun. Whether it is a common cold, or something more serious like strep throat, taking time out of our life to heal can be frustrating (and painful)! Heading to the doctor for every sniffle and sneeze can get costly, and usually isn't necessary. In many cases, Nature has the cure.

At the first sign of any illness, give your immune system a boost by mixing the juice of one lemon, an equal amount of raw honey, a one-inch piece of fresh ginger, and 4-5 garlic cloves. I have found it best to throw them all in a small food processor, but it works just as well if you simply crush/grate the ginger and garlic. Take one tablespoon every 3-4 hours for three days. This mixture can help you avoid taking prescription antibiotics that can cause severe side effects, or that upset the delicate balance of good bacteria in the body.

A common complaint through the warm months of the year is red, itchy eyes due to allergies, irritants or infection. Eyebright is my go-to herb for any eye issues. When mixed with calendula, chamomile and burdock root, combating eye issues is a simple process. Combine equal amounts of these herbs, then add 1 tablespoon of the herb blend to 1 cup of hot (not boiling) water and let steep for 20-30 minutes. Strain well, then use the tea as an eyewash several times a day until the issue is resolved. You can also soak a cotton ball in the tea and place it on the eyelids. Let sit for 20-30 minutes.

Ear infections are common complaints that are easily managed using natural remedies. Mix ¼ cup olive oil with 5 drops each of lavender and tea tree oil to kill infection, ease pain and inflammation, and help release any water or wax that has built up in the ear canal. During the summer months when you can find mullein in bloom, gather some of the tiny yellow flowers. Let them dry for a day or two, then place them in a small jar. Add enough olive oil to completely cover the flowers. Place the mixture in a cool, dark place and shake well daily for 4-5 weeks. Strain the mixture, add the above essential oil blend, and you have a powerful tool at your fingertips for any type of ear issues. When you need to use it, warm it gently by running it under hot tap water, then place 3 drops in the effected ear. Seal it in with a small bit of cotton. Never place your herbal oils in the microwave to warm them, as this destroys the beneficial characteristics.

Sinus infections can be extremely painful, and tend to linger. At the first sign of pain or inflammation, a Neti pot is the fastest, most effective treatment. Combine 2 cups of warm, distilled water and ½ teaspoon of sea salt. For a bit of extra healing power, add 1/8 teaspoon of golden seal powder. Mix well. Repeat twice daily.

Of course, the best line of defense is a good offense. You can ward off many illnesses by eating a healthy diet that includes daily servings of fresh fruits and vegetables, and plenty of clean water. Don't forget to spend some time outdoors. Fresh air, sunshine and exercise help rid the body of toxins, provide Vitamin D and oxygen to the body, and helps speed healing from illnesses of every variety.

81 BEFORE YOU BURN THOSE LEAVES

I was sitting next to a sweet friend at a meeting recently, and she told me she had been stuffing leaves into bags for the "Leaf man." That of course caught my attention, and she went on to explain a leaf buyer comes to town periodically to buy walnut and sassafras leaves.

That made perfect sense to me, as I'm well aware of the medicinal properties of these plants. I've even written several articles about a home-based weed-a-ceutical business opportunity right here in the Ozarks, where native plants abound and are free for the picking.

Walnut Leaves

Black walnuts, the type that we find here at home, have about the same amounts of calories, protein, vitamins and minerals as English walnuts, but are higher in arginine and selenium, but lower in Omega 3 fatty acids. Black walnuts are definitely more expensive than the English variety, and they literally grow on trees here in the Ozarks.

Throughout Europe, walnut leaves are popular in treating eczema and swelling of the eyes. Walnut leaves can be moistened, and "bruised" to release the active ingredients, then applied to areas of eczema, or applied to the external eyelid for swelling and inflammation. A tincture can also be made with the fresh or dried leaves, and stored in a cool place for later use. In addition to treating eczema, (an itchy, patchy recurrent rash), walnut leaves are also used to treat ringworm and acne. For treating acne, the leaves are used to make a face wash by steeping the leaves in hot water as you would when making tea. The solution works as both an astringent and an antibacterial skin cleanser. For ringworm, apply a walnut leaf compress to the affected area. A walnut leaf foot soak has also been reported as a treatment for athlete's foot.

Black walnut leaf tea sells for about $2.00 per ounce on Amazon. Customer reviews show it is used to treat pinworms in children, an effect that can be attributed to the juglone content in the tea.

Those fleshy green walnut husks? They are valuable, too, rich in fruit acids and minerals, and can be used to make a hair rinse to darken hair.

Sassafras Leaves

Do you like gumbo? Sassafras leaves are essential as a thickening and seasoning agent in Cajun cooking, making them very valuable, and in high demand in certain regions of the country.

In addition to their use in cooking, sassafras leaves have properties that can decrease pain and speed healing. The leaves can be applied as a poultice to a wound, reducing pain and inflammation. Sassafras contains safrole, a blood thinner that works by decreasing platelet activity. This is a beneficial effect, because it helps to bring oxygenated blood to the area where the poultice is applied, helping to rebuild damaged tissue.

Anywhere else in this beautiful country of ours, burning leaves is appropriate. When in the Ozarks, think twice, because you just might be burning money.

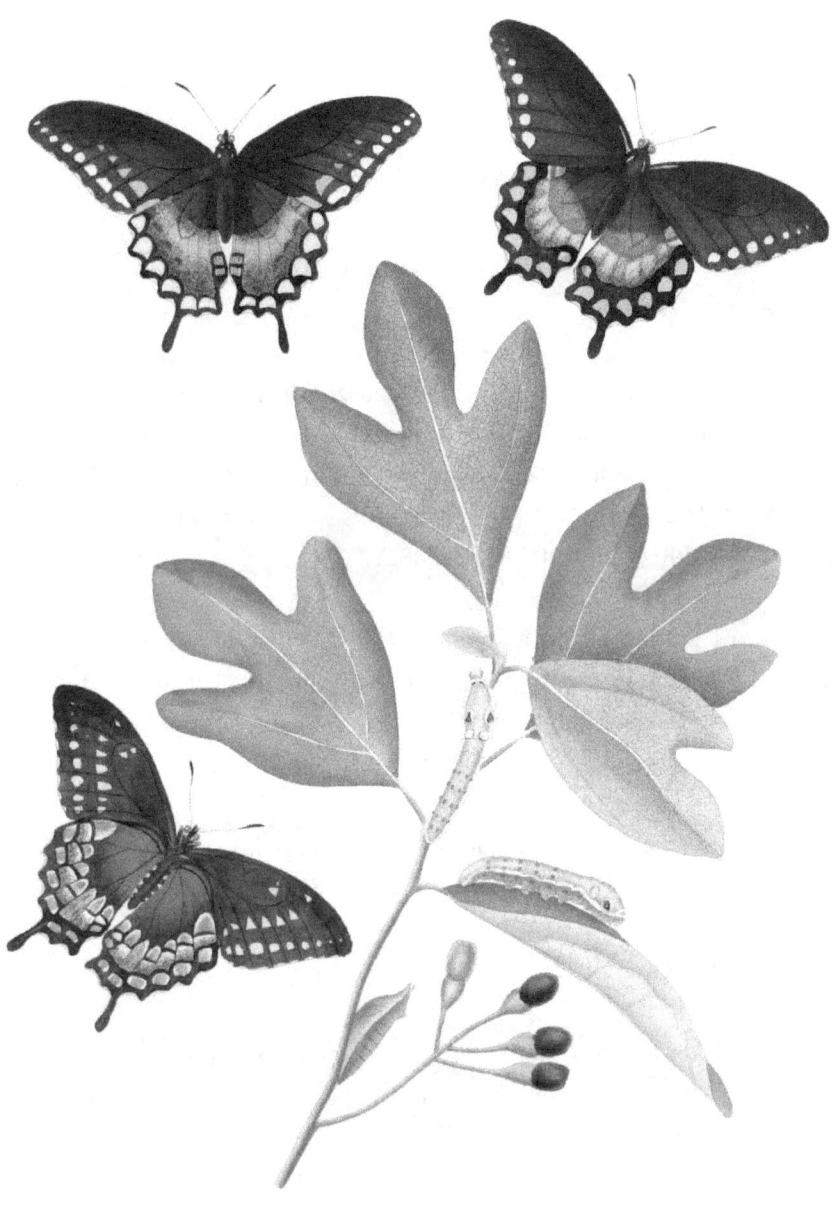

Sassafras is a host plant for the Spicebush Swallowtail. Abbot, John, 1751-1840 (artist).

82 THE TRUTH ABOUT CBD OIL :WHAT YOU MAY NOT KNOW ABOUT CANNABIS

By: Candice Schwien

*Just a note: I am not endorsing the legalization of marijuana (Cannabis) in any shape, form or fashion. I am also not opposing cannabis. I am merely trying to share the knowledge and information I have found on the benefits of the STUDIED compounds within the PLANT when they are used CORRECTLY and RESPONSIBLY.

Why am I writing about cannabis? Well, I am a health enthusiast, so when I find something might have health benefits, I research it. I have thoroughly researched cannabis, and its uses. What I found was incredibly interesting. And I wanted to share it with you.

Cannabis is a plant, which means it can be used naturally for health, in the right ways, using the right strains, under the right circumstances.

First, what is Cannabis?

Cannabis is a flowering plant from the Cannabaceae family. There are co untless species, but the three most well-known are cannabis sativa, cannabis indica, and cannabis ruderalis.

Cannabis is widely known for its uses as hemp fiber, hemp oils, its use in medicine, and as a recreational drug. In fact, in history, it was once illegal NOT to grow hemp because of its great uses. It was even considered currency at one time.

When hemp is used for paper and rope, or for hemp oil, they use a strain that is bred for high fiber. And they use almost every part of the plant, if not all of it.

But when it's used as a recreational drug, they are using a different strain, bred especially for high THC (Tetrahydrocannabinol-the hallucinogenic in marijuana). Now, THC does have health benefits in very small doses or used equally with CBD. However; when it is HEATED (dried and then smoked) it is EXTREMELY harmful to one's health. It dries the body from the inside out, and with our bodies being made up of 70% water, we need to stay hydrated.

The flower buds when dried are usually known as marijuana or hash and used as a drug. This is what became illegal in most parts of the world. It's illegal to grow or possess cannabis for sale or personal use. (This is all the media covers, which is why so many people don't know it's NOT illegal to use CBD oil).

Cannabinoids

All cannabis plants produce chemical compounds known as cannabinoids. These cannabinoids produce different mental and physical effects when consumed and act on cannabinoid receptors inside cells that alter neurotransmitter release in the brain. Ligands for these receptor proteins include endocannabinoids, that are naturally produced in the human body.

Endocannabinoids are neurotransmitters that bind to cannabinoid receptors and proteins that are then expressed throughout the nervous system. They are found all throughout the body, in the brain and all the organs..

So, the endocannabinoid system REGULATES or BALANCES physiological and cognitive (thinking) processes. Which means it regulates the body's internal balance, including appetite, pain, mood, memory, and fertility (pregnancy pre and postnatal development). And it balances or mediates the pharmacological effects of cannabis.

The ECS (endocannabinoid system) also balances the physiological and Cognitive effects of voluntary exercise "runner's high," like the release of euphoria when you go for a short run, making you feel happy. The euphoria also causes the pain receptors to lessen, which is why you don't always feel the pain until the "high" is gone.

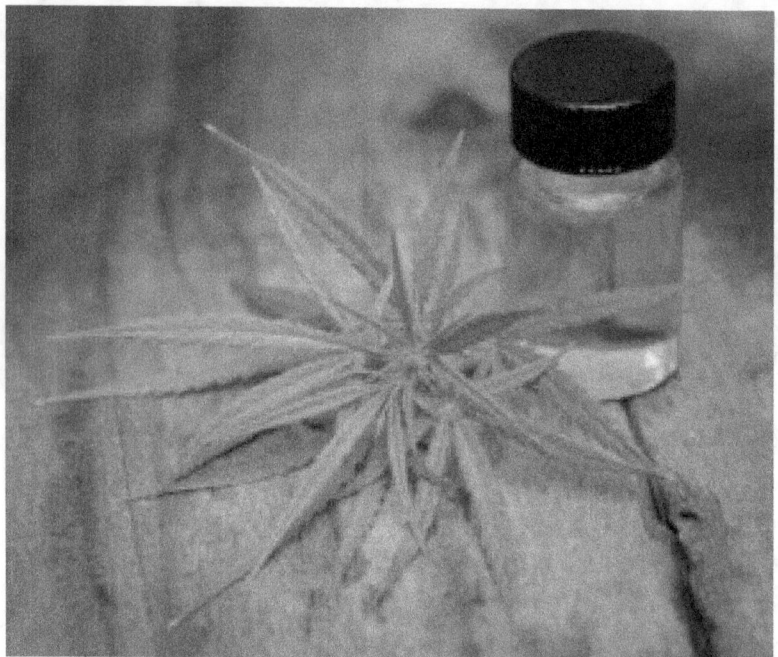

Continued next week...

83 THE BENEFITS OF CBD OIL – PART 2

By: Candice Schwien

The benefits of CBD oil are still being studied, and since there are so many amazing benefits I am not going to list them all here, but CBD Oil can:

1) Relieve Chronic Pain

CBD Oil can relieve chronic pain associated with diseases like fibromyalgia, multiple sclerosis, and cancer. It also relieves neuropathic pain. Because CBD oil does not cause dependencies like morphine or other intense painkillers it has become the first choice for any persons wanting to avoid modern medicine and opioids.

Most Opioids are synthetic, where CBD oil is natural. Opioids do not work with your body to relieve pain which is why they are so highly addictive and usually have to be taken long term. So, while they dull the pain short term, they cause addiction, and since they do not work with the body's natural system they cause horrible long-lasting side effects.

2) Diabetes

CBD Oil can be used to lower type 1 diabetes in early stages. There are still several studies ongoing for the treatment of diabetes.

3) Epilepsy/Seizures

CBD Oil has been studied to improve treatment-resistant epilepsy in children. 84% experienced reduced frequency along with better moods, increased alertness, and better sleep after 3 months of treatment. 39% of children had more than 50% reduction of seizures altogether. The study also showed that 7 out of 8 children had a more improved state of disease altogether after the study ended.

4) Relieves Rheumatoid Arthritis

CBD Oil has been studied to decrease the pain associated with rheumatoid arthritis. Because of its anti-inflammatory property, it showed decreases in joint destruction and slowed disease progression.

5) Reduces Stress, Anxiety, & Depression

CBD Oil is probably most noted for its ability to reduce anxiety. Over 24% of the US population suffers from anxiety or depression. Our bodies have a fight or flight tendency when introduced to stress. With the modern day we live in, we are almost always in contact with stress in one way or another. This causes us to be in an anxious state almost constantly. This state of anxiety affects every single organ in our body. If we live in a continued state of anxiety or stress, it affects our health in major ways. CBD Oil has been shown to reduce that stress and help create a more peaceful state of mind. It has been shown to greatly help those suffering from OCD (Obsessive Compulsive Disorder), PTSD(Post Traumatic Stress Disorder), & Social Anxiety.

6) Fights drug-resistant bacteria

CBD Oil will fight modern day 'Superbugs' that are becoming resistant to modern antioxidants. CBD Oil inhibits the cells causing the bacteria and destroys them.

7) Reduces Autoimmune Disease

CBD oil for autoimmune disease is still being studied further, but it has been shown to reduce the pain of autoimmune disease. CBD Oil helps the body regulate or balance which stops the immune system's overactive response to normal body tissues or substances. In other words, it stops the body from attacking itself.

8) Acne, eczema, & psoriasis

CBD oil has been found to decrease skin secretions helping with overactive oil glands. It also stabilizes the skins pH, reducing itching, burning, and inflammation from eczema. CBD oil also has anti-inflammatory and antiproliferative properties that help against the symptoms of psoriasis.

9) Heart Health

CBD Oil has been studied to cause dilation of the arteries around the heart and protect damaged blood vessels. It also has been shown to reduce the size of damage to the heart or brain. It helps reduce the heart rate and blood pressure in response to stress as well. And it was also noted to influence white blood cell functions.

10) IBS & Digestive issues

The studies of CBD Oil have found that it blocks the mechanisms of spinal, gastrointestinal and peripheral nerves that cause pain associated with IBS (irritable bowel syndrome). The resins and oils in CBD oil help treat and relieve gastrointestinal distress. By preventing inflammation in the digestive tract and intestines, CBD oil relieves the pain and relaxes the muscles to prevent spasms. It also treats Crohn's disease and colitis. CBD oils help calm the immune pathways and overactivity. It's been shown to help with nausea and vomiting.

84 INCLINED BED THERAPY

How you sleep matters. If you ever gone to bed with a cold and cough, you figure out quickly that sleeping on two pillows helps your breathing. Night shift nurses who finally lay down to sleep after their shift find they suddenly have to get up to urinate every few hours as fluids trapped in their legs slowly return to the kidneys after the nurse has been on her feet all night. Of course, if you have swelling of your legs and feet, your health care professional encourages you to elevate your legs when you can.

At some point in history, people decided they should sleep on a flat surface. This wasn't always the case, as ancient beds were tilted at least a 5 degree angle in many cultures. Archeological artifacts from Egypt include inclined beds, with the head on these beds 6 inches higher than the foot end. Animals also prefer to sleep with their head in a raised position, as you've probably noticed with the family dog.

Several studies have found that sleeping at a 3.5 to 5 degree incline is beneficial. Not talking about a hospital bed that bends in the middle with the head of the bed raised, the entire bed should be on a slope, and accomplished with putting blocks under the head of the bed, raising it approximately six inches. Benefits include improved blood circulation and breathing function, accelerated metabolism, and enhanced neurologic and immune functions. Other conditions that may be helped with inclined bed therapy include diabetes, glaucoma, migraines, multiple sclerosis, sleep apnea, acid reflux, edema, and varicose veins, as noted below.

Andrew K. Fletcher is credited with discovering the benefits of inclined bed therapy. He likened the activity of water moving up through the trunk of a tree via the roots to the flow of fluids through the human body. In order to see how gravity and the flow of water affects the human body, he tried placing bricks under the head of his bed to raise it. His wife saw the benefits first, when her varicose veins improved tremendously within the space of a month.

Migraines

Sleeping on an incline affects intracranial pressure. Research by a medical anthropologist showed people with migraines were able to eliminate their migraines within a short period of time by sleeping with their heads raised. In fact, in the neurological ICU, nurses are trained to elevate the head of the patients bed when intracranial pressure becomes too high.

Acid Reflux

Many people suffer from acid reflux, or GERD. Often the only time symptoms occur is when laying down in bed at night, when corrosive stomach acid refluxes up into your esophagus, causing pain that feels like acid is eating away at your tissue, which it is. The stomach lining is designed to withstand this acid, but the delicate tissues of the esophagus aren't. Inclined bed therapy will not cure this condition, but it can help keep gastric acid in the right place, your stomach, when you are trying to sleep.

Frequent night Urination

If getting up frequently at night to urinate plagues you, try raising the head of your bed. Many anecdotal reports attest to people getting better sleep because they are sleeping at least six hours at a stretch instead of having to get up every two hours to urinate.

Edema

While elevating swollen lower extremities can definitely lessen edema, many people with chronic edema have seen improvement with inclined bed therapy with the head of the bed elevated. Improvement has also been seen with hemorrhoids.

If you have any of the problems listed above, why not give inclined bed therapy a try?

85 CHIA

Who didn't have a chia pet when they were growing up? It turns out these tiny black seeds are more than a novelty item. First, the tiny "seeds" are actually dried fruit. Chia seeds are rich in protein, fiber, vitamins and minerals; especially calcium, magnesium, iron and zinc. They are excellent anti-oxidants, rich in Omega-3 fatty acids like those found in fish.

Medical benefits of chia seeds include anti-inflammatory, antidiabetic and fever reducing properties, and have been found to specifically slow the growth of cancer cells without harming normal cells in the body.

Nutrition

Chia seeds are classified as a functional food, one that provides health benefits beyond just nutrition. The Latin name is *Salvia hispanica*, and chia is native to Central America where the seeds served as a staple food in the Mayan and Aztec diets. They can easily be added to many food products, soups, stews, baked goods, etc. to enhance the Omega-3 and fiber content. They are an excellent source of linoleic fatty acid, an essential fatty acid that decreases blood pressure, among other things. Chia seeds are higher in protein at 16.5% than other grains, including wheat, corn, rice barley and amaranth.

Chia seeds are a great source of dietary fiber, promoting regular bowel movements and helping in weight loss due to a feeling of satiety that reduces appetite. Soluble fiber in chia seeds absorbs water, forming a gel in the stomach that promotes probiotics in the gut. As an added benefit, chia seeds are gluten free, making them safe for gluten free diets. Replacement of wheat in bread with chia seeds and/or chia flour reduces saturated fatty acids in the completed product.

Several studies have shown that chia seeds are very helpful for Type 2 diabetics. Subjects consuming 37 grams of chia seeds daily showed lower blood pressure and reduced pro-inflammatory markers and decreased tendency to blood clots. Another study documented a significant decrease in waist circumference in healthy persons after chia supplementation for just one month. In animal studies, chia seeds lowered lipid and triglyceride levels in the blood, raised the level of HDL (good cholesterol) and decreased fat deposits around internal organs.

Chia seeds contain several valuable components, including caffeic acid, rosemarinic acid and quercetin, known as a natural antihistamine that relieves seasonal and food allergies, controls blood pressure and helps with pain. Caffeic acid has anti-oxidant and anti-inflammatory properties, while rosmarinic acid has antioxidant, astringent, anti-inflammatory, anticlot, anti-cancer, antibacterial and antiviral properties. Chia seeds provide all these benefits in just one source.

Precautions

While chia seeds are non-toxic and gluten free, they can cause problems in people with swallowing problems due to the fact they can expand greatly by absorbing up to twenty-seven times their weight in water. Dr. Rebecca Rawl, from Carolinas Medical Center in Charlotte, N.C. cautions "patients with a history of known esophageal strictures should be cautioned that chia seeds should only be consumed when they have had the ability to fully expand in liquid prior to ingestion." In fact, a 39-year-old man with a history of swallowing problems ran into trouble after eating a tablespoon of dry chia seeds with a glass of water. The seeds swelled in his esophagus, and he began choking. Doctors who examined him in a nearby emergency room found a gel of wet chia seeds was blocking his esophagus. The blockage was cleared with medical help, but clearly eating dry chia seeds should be avoided.

238

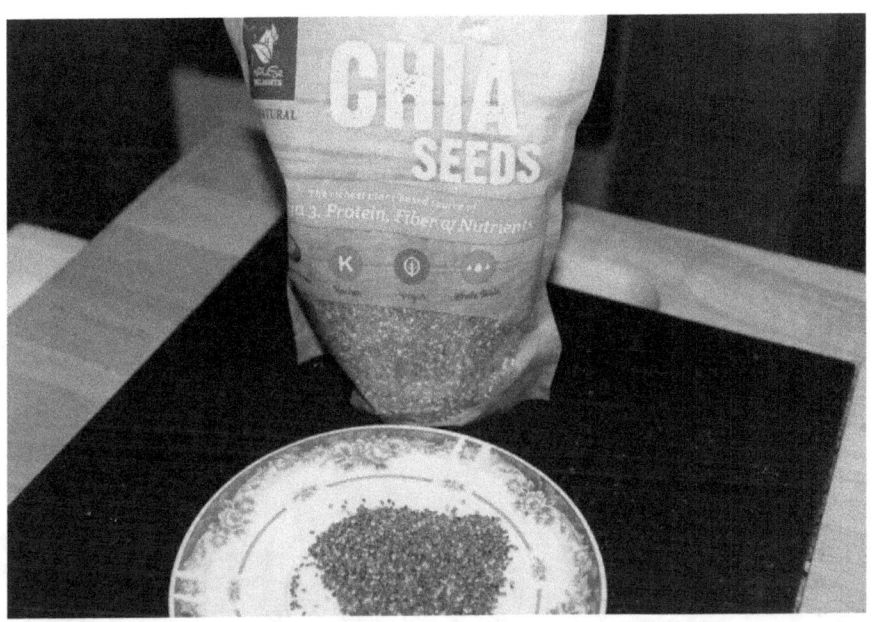

Chia seeds are actually tiny dried fruits.

Marie Lasater

INDEX

niacin deficiency, 1–2
nose, 71, 215

O
obesity, 21, 40, 92, 95, 133–34, 166–67, 180, 202
obesity prevention, 95, 134
Obsessive Compulsive Disorder, 232
opiate withdrawal, 191
opioid receptors, 191
opioids, 189, 191, 210, 231
osteoarthritis, 85, 133
outbreaks, 5
  blue tongue virus, 128
  cold sore, 101
  herpes, 220
ovarian syndrome, 53
ox-eye daisy, 81–82
Ozarks, 81, 83, 94, 198–99, 205, 210, 220, 225–26

P
pain
  arthritis, 60
  block, 24
  chest, 207
  hip, 124
  jaw, 207
  joint, 9, 100
  leg, 121
  menstrual, 85
  nerve, 37
  neuropathic, 231
Paracelsus, 149
paralysis, 30, 51
Parkinson's Disease, 6, 70, 76
peptic ulcer, 95
phlegm, 117, 194
Pine-sol, 32, 78
Plantago Lanceolata, 117
plantain, 103, 117, 199

U

ulcers, 33, 46, 117
ultraviolet, 152, 167
ultraviolet protection, 167

V

vaccines, 4–5, 30, 157–58
  swine flu, 30–31
vision, 169–72
  improving, 171
vision loss, 169, 171
vision restoration techniques, popular, 172
Vitamin B3, 1–2
vitamin D3, 152
vomiting, 60, 106, 156, 183, 209, 233

W

weight loss, 40, 60, 72, 92–93, 167, 218, 237
white clover, 75–77
White clover honey, 75
White Nursery, George O., 27, 96, 219
Wild lettuce, 210
Wild Sweet Potatoes, 106
wine, 94, 147, 217
wintergreen, 182, 215
wintergreen plant, 182
worry, 16, 78, 164
wound healing, 84–85, 128, 220
wounds, deep, 84, 185

Z

zinc, 89, 104, 237

ABOUT THE AUTHOR

Marie Lasater has always been interested in health and natural cures. At the time of this writing, she has left the field of nursing and is serving as elected County Coroner, and is a board-certified medicolegal death investigator - a role that melds well with her passion for research. The chapters in this book and the preceding two books in the series are taken from her locally syndicated column. She follows in the footsteps of a distant cousin, Francis Marion Beynon, who wrote a similar column from 1912 - 1917 entitled "The Country Homemaker's Page," which served as a platform for the writer's political views, and helped to secure women's right to vote and hold office in Canada.

www.ingramcontent.com/pod-product-compliance
Lightning Source LLC
Chambersburg PA
CBHW060452290526
45791CB00001B/81